Viva Voce in

Oral
Medicine and
Radiology

Viva Voce in
Oral
Medicine and
Radiology

Tapasya Vaibhav Karemore MDS

Associate Professor
Department of Oral Medicine and Radiology
VSPM Dental College, Nagpur
Maharashtra

Preeti Chawla Arora MDS

Associate Professor and Subject In-charge
SGRD Dental College
Amritsar

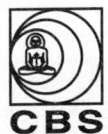

CBS

CBS Publishers & Distributors Pvt Ltd

New Delhi • Bengaluru • Chennai • Kochi • Kolkata • Mumbai
Bhopal • Bhubaneswar • Hyderabad • Jharkhand • Nagpur • Patna • Pune • Uttarakhand • Dhaka (Bangladesh)

Viva Voce in
Oral
Medicine and
Radiology

ISBN: 978-93-88527-74-3

Copyright © Authors and Publisher

First Edition: 2019

Published by Satish Kumar Jain and produced by Varun Jain for

CBS Publishers & Distributors Pvt Ltd

4819/XI Prahlad Street, 24 Ansari Road, Daryaganj, New Delhi 110 002, India.

Ph: 23289259, 23266861, 23266867   Fax: 011-23243014
Website: www.cbspd.com   e-mail: delhi@cbspd.com; cbspubs@airtelmail.in.

Corporate Office: 204 FIE, Industrial Area, Patparganj, Delhi 110 092
Ph: 4934 4934   Fax: 4934 4935
    e-mail: publishing@cbspd.com; publicity@cbspd.com

Branches

- **Bengaluru:** Seema House 2975, 17th Cross, K.R. Road, Banasankari 2nd Stage, Bengaluru 560 070, Karnataka
  Ph: +91-80-26771678/79   Fax: +91-80-26771680   e-mail: bangalore@cbspd.com
- **Chennai:** 7, Subbaraya Street, Shenoy Nagar, Chennai 600 030, Tamil Nadu
  Ph: +91-44-26680620, 26681266   Fax: +91-44-42032115   e-mail: chennai@cbspd.com
- **Kochi:** 42/1325, 1326, Power House Road, Opposite KSEB Power House, Ernakulam 682 018, Kochi, Kerala
  Ph: +91-484-4059061-65   Fax: +91-484-4059065   e-mail: kochi@cbspd.com
- **Kolkata:** 6/B, Ground Floor, Rameswar Shaw Road, Kolkata-700 014, West Bengal
  Ph: +91-33-22891126, 22891127, 22891128   e-mail: kolkata@cbspd.com
- **Mumbai:** 83-C, Dr E Moses Road, Worli, Mumbai-400018, Maharashtra
  Ph: +91-22-24902340/41   Fax: +91-22-24902342   e-mail: mumbai@cbspd.com

Representatives

• **Bhopal**	0-8319310552	• **Bhubaneswar**	0-9911037372
• **Hyderabad**	0-9885175004	• **Jharkhand**	0-9811541605
• **Nagpur**	0-9421945513	• **Patna**	0-9334159340
• **Pune**	0-9623451994	• **Uttarakhand**	0-9716462459
• **Dhaka (Bangladesh)**	01912-0034853		

Printed at Mudrak, Noida, UP, India

Preface

It is a moment of pleasure to introduce a book in oral medicine and radiology based on *viva voce* examination. Oral medicine and radiology is a vast subject and it needs thorough preparation of any subject to excel. The students sometimes find it difficult to prepare especially for *viva* examination. The concept has been conceived to help the students for preparing the subject well, facing every question in the examination and learning the subject from every corner. We have tried to incorporate all the topics in the subject in terms of *viva* questions and used tables and diagrams wherever necessary. We sincerely hope that undergraduates will find this book rewarding and informative. We solicit valuable suggestions and constructive feedback from the readers of this book to enable us to incorporate them in future editions. You can send your feedback to *tapasyamds@gmail.com* and *dr.preets@gmail.com*

Dear students....wish you all the best!!!

Tapasya Vaibhav Karemore
Preeti Chawla Arora

Contents

Section II

Radiology

Introduction

Assessment of student's knowledge has various dimensions in Indian education set up. *Viva voce* is one of the commonly practiced examinations amongst them since health profession schools were established. *Viva voce* is a form of assessment, which was traditionally chosen for its flexibility and potential for the testing of cognitive skills, which are closely associated with medical practice. To analyze validity, feasibility and reliability of viva, many academicians have studied every angle of it. It was suggested that, to make it more standardized, including a large number of questions and encompassing widest possible content would help to maximize the validity of viva as an assessment tool.

Considering the need of time and suggestions by students, an attempt is made to produce a guide for revising *Oral Medicine and Radiology*. Though it is never meant to replace textbooks but can help in many ways to recollect at the last hours and regain the confidence. It is good to read textbook followed by this guide for better retention of the topic learnt. We are sure that this book will change your perception for the subject and your apprehension of revising the vast course in limited time.

Best wishes!!

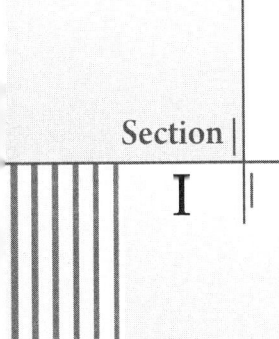

Oral Medicine

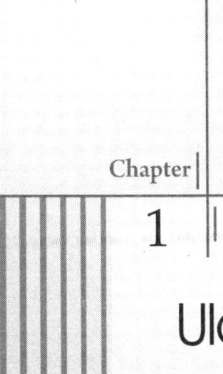

Ulcerative Vesiculobullous Lesions

Q1. Define ulcer, vesicle, macule, papule, pustule, plaque, bulla and nodule with examples.

Ans.
- **Ulcer:** A defect in the epithelium; it is well circumscribed depressed lesion over which epidermal layers has been lost with molecular necrosis. It is also described as break in the continuity of epithelium due to molecular necrosis.

  For example, aphthous ulcer, traumatic ulcer, herpetic ulcer.

- **Macule:** Well circumscribed, flat lesions that are noticeable because of their change from normal skin color. May be red due to presence of vascular lesions or inflammation, or pigmented due to presence of melanin, hemosiderin, drugs.

  For example, haemangioma.

- **Papule:** Solid lesions, raised above the skin surface that are smaller than 1 cm diameter.

  For example, erythema multiforme, rubella, lupus erythematous.

- **Plaque:** Solid raised lesions that are over 1 cm in diameter; they are larger papules

  For example, leukoplakia.

- **Bulla:** Elevated blisters like lesions containing clear fluid that are over 1 cm in diameter.

For example, pemphigus.

- **Nodule:** These lesions are present deep in the dermis and the epidermis can be easily moved over them.
  For example, fibroma.
- **Pustule:** Raised lesions containing purulent material.

Q2. What are erosions?

Ans. Moist red lesions often caused by the rupture of vesicles or bullae as well as trauma.
Example: Oral lichen planus.

Q3. Give examples of ulcers caused by viral infection.

Ans. • Herpes simplex infection
- Herpangina
- Measles (paramyxovirus—Koplik's spots)
- Herpes zoster
- Hand–foot and mouth disease
- Infectious mononucleosis
- HIV-AIDS

Q4. Give example of ulcers caused by bacterial infection.

Ans. • Syphilis
- Tuberculosis
- ANUG
- Gonorrhea
- Leprosy
- Actinomycosis
- Noma
- Scarlet fever
- Diphtheria

Q5. Give examples of ulcers caused by fungal infections.

Ans. • Histoplamosis
- Blastomycosis
- Mucormycosis
- Cryptococcosis

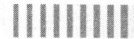

Q6. Types of edges in different types of ulcers.

Ans. • Gumma punched out
  • Healing/venous ulcersloping
  • Malignant ulcer rolled out
  • Rodent ulcer (basal cell carcinoma)—beaded
  • Tuberculosis—undermined

Q7. Ulcers associated with immunologic defects:

Ans. • Pemphigus
  • Cicatricial pemphigoid
  • Bullous pemphigoid
  • Dermatitis herpetiformis
  • Linear IgA disease
  • Epidermolysis bullosa acquisita
  • Erythema multiforme

Q8. Acute multiple vesiculobullous lesions:

Ans. • Herpes virus infection
  • Aphthous ulcer
  • Primary herpes simplex virus infections
  • Coxsackievirus infections
  • Varicella zoster virus infection
  • Erythema multiforme
  • Contact allergic stomatitis
  • Oral ulcers secondary to cancer chemotherapy
  • Acute necrotizing ulcerative gingivitis

Q9. Chronic multiple vesiculobullous lesions:

Ans. • Pemphigus vulgaris and vegetans
  • Bullous pemphigoid
  • Mucous membrane pemphigoid
  • Erosive lichen planus
  • Linear IgA disease
  • Chronic herpes simplex infection in cancer chemo-
    therapy, immunocompromised states and HIV.

Q10. Lesions associated with single ulcers.

Ans.
- Histoplasmosis
- Blastomycosis
- Mucormycosis
- Syphilitic ulcer
- TB ulcer
- Malignant ulcer
- Traumatic ulcer

Q11. What are characteristic features of herpetic ulcers?

Ans.
- **SRSS:** Smooth, round, shallow and symmetrical
- **Drops of dew appearance**
- **Moon crater appearance**
- Associated with gingivostomatitis
- Age 6 months to 6 years

Q12. Which are DNA viruses?

Ans. There are 6 viruses: HSV 1, HSV 2, HZV, cytomegalovirus, EBV, HHV.

Q13. Which are RNA viruses?

Ans. Coxsackievirus, HIV and hepatitis B.

Q14. Why is aspirin contraindicated in primary HSV?

Ans. Reye's syndrome (liver damage in children)

Q15. HSV is associated with which ganglions?

Ans.
- Trigeminal ganglion
- Dorsal root ganglion

Q16. Treatment of primary HSV infection:

Ans.
- Doses: Topical acyclovir
- If systemic then, acyclovir 200 mg, 5 times daily
- For children—15 mg/kg body weight
- Liquid intake and topical anaesthetics.

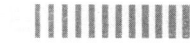

Q17. Various HSV related lesions:

Ans. • Primary herpes simplex infection

• Recurrent herpes labialis (Recrudescent HSV)

• Herpetic whitlow

• Herpetic barbae

• Herpetic paronychia

• Herpetic gladiatorum

Q18. What is Coxsackievirus infection?

Ans. • Term "Coxsackie" is from a town in New York (name from where it was 1st discovered)

• Coxsackie group A lesions are herpangina (*coxsackie A 6, 8, 10*)

• Hand, foot and mouth disease *coxsackie A16*

• Acute lymphonodular pharyngitis (*coxsackie A10*) and rarely mumps like parotitis.

Q19. Lab diagnosis of HSV:

Ans. • Cytology—syncytium formation

• Viral isolation

• Antibody titers (convalescent sera-4 fold rise = Acute infection)

• Co-Paul test

Q20. Dose of steroids in herpes simplex infection:

Ans. Steroids are contraindicated.

Q21. Characteristics of herpangina:

Ans. Epidemic—June to October

• Mainly young

• Less severe symptoms than HSV

Q22. Differences between HSV and Herpangina
Ans.

HSV	Herpangina
1. Severe	1. Milder
2. Non-epidemic	2. Epidemic
3. Anterior portion of mouth esp. gingiva	3. Posterior portion e.g. palate
4. Gingivitis	4. No-gingivitis
5. larger SSSR	5. Smaller lesions Macule- papule-vesicle-ulcer
6. DNA virus	6. RNA virus
7. HSV	7. A4 Coxsackie
8. Cytology shows multi-nucleated Tzanck cells	8. Absence of multi-nucleated giant cells
9. Management: Specific antiviral for 1^0 HSV	9. Self limiting and supportive treatment needed

Q23. Difference between HSV and EM.
Ans.

HSV	EM
1. SSSR*	1. LIDB*
2. Prodromal symptoms (period—2 to 8 days) Fever before	2. Fever may sometimes accompany (no prodromal symptoms) Sudden acute explosive onset
3. Age–primary 6 month to 6 yrs	3. Age—younger adults
4. Etiology–viral	4. Hypersensitivity reaction
5. Marginal gingivitis	5. No gingival involvement Lips prominently involved
6. Cervical lymphadenopathy -+nt	6. -nt
7. No target/bull's eye lesion	7. Target/bull's eye lesion

*SSSR: Smooth, round, shallow, symmetrical
*LIDB: Large, irregular, deep and bleeding

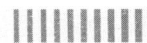

Q24. Difference between HSV and HZV.

Ans.

HSV	HZV
1. Lesions do not heal by scarring	1. Scarring +nt
2. No osteonecrosis	2. In severe—osteonecrosis
3. HSV – 1° and 2° RHL and RIOH	3. VZ – 1° chickenpox and HZ
4. Bilateral	4. Unilateral
5. Prodromal symptoms; fever, malaise No pain only tingling.	5. Prodromal symptoms shooting pain, burning paraesthesia and tenderness along the nerve area—C_3, T_5, L_1, L_2 No H/o fever
6. Cytology—Tzanck cells	6. Non-specific cytology
7. Rx acyclovir 200 mg 5 times a day	7. Rx acyclovir 800 mg 5 times a day

Q25. Infections caused by varicella zoster virus.

Ans. Primary-chickenpox (varicella) which remains dormant in dorsal root ganglia and can reactivate in immuno-suppressive states to causes unilateral vesicles and pain along the course of the nerve causing secondary infection, i.e herpes zoster/Shingles. It involves the trigeminal nerve and C3, T5, L1 and L2. These vesicles resemble **Dew Drops on Rose Petal**.

Q26. Complications of herpes zoster.

Ans. • Unilateral pain in herpes zoster without lesions is called zoster sine herpete/zoster sine eruption)
• Hutchinson sign: It is cutaneous zoster infection of the side of tip of nose.
• Syndrome associated: Ramsay Hunt syndrome [triad of ipsilateral facial paralysis, ear pain and vesicles on face on the ear is typical presentation]
• Post-herpetic neuralgia (unilateral pain lingering for more than a month)

- Blindness secondary to corneal scarring in ophthalmic division involvement.
- Pulpal necrosis
- Internal root resorption
- Osteonecrosis and exfoliation of teeth
- Recurrent episodes of HZ may be indicative of some underlying malignancy.
- Treatment–800 mg acyclovir 5 times daily

Q27 **Only indication of corticosteroids in viral infections of oral cavity.**

Ans. Corticosteroids may be given only in few cases of herpes zoster to prevent the risk of post-herpetic neuralgia.

Q28. Types of erythema multiforme:

Ans. 1. EM major—more than 10% skin involvement.

2. EM minor—less than 10% skin involvement.

Q29. Etiology of erythema multiforme:

Ans. • Infection, particularly HSV, mycoplasma, pneumonia
- Drug reactions to NSAIDs, anticonvulsants
- Oral EM precipitated by benzoic acid
- HSV (concurrent RHL)

Q30. Characterstic features of ulcers associated with erythema multiforme.

Ans. • Large, irregular, deep and bleeding (LIDB).
- Crustation on lips.
- **Target iris/bull's eye** lesions.
- No prodomal symptoms and sudden, acute explosive onset

Q31. Complications of erythema multiforme.

Ans. • Stevens-Johnson syndrome (ocular and genital lesions)
- Lyell's disease/TEN (toxic epidermal necrolysis)

Q32. Treatment of erythema multiforme.

Ans. 30–50 mg prednisolone, if associated with then HSV acyclovir 800–1200 mg

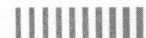

Q33. What is contact stomatitis?

Ans. Two types
- *Stomatitis venenata:* Allergy to food stuffs/coloring agents/cinnamon/mango/chewing gum/cosmetics
- *Stomatitis medicamentosa:* Allergy to medicaments/dental materials.
  - Diagnosis: Patch test
  - Treatment by topical steroids and antiallergic.

Q34. What is ANUG?

Ans. 1. Other names: Trench mouth (it gets its name from World War I, as it affected soldiers in the trenches)
2. Vincent's angina (after the name of French physician Henri Vincent)

Q35. Etiology of ANUG.

Ans. • Anaerobic bacteria particularly *Fusobacteria, Spirochaeta* (Treponema) sp.
- Smoking
- Debiliated patient under stress
- Poor oral hygiene
- Nutritional deficiencies
- Immunodeficiency (e.g. HIV/AIDS, use of immuno-suppressive drugs)
- Sleep deprivation

Q36. Characterstic features of ANUG.

Ans. • Punched out necrotic ulcers without
  - Pseudomembrane of interdental gingiva
  - Woody sensation of teeth

Q37. Necrosis of tissues seen in which conditions?

Ans. • ANUG/NOMA
  - Necrotizing sialometaplasia
  - Leukemic ulcers
  - Cyclic neutropenia

- Agranulocytosis
- Chédiak-Higashi syndrome

Q38. Types of angina (*refers* to choking sensation).

Ans. • Vincent's angina
- Angina pectoris
- Diphtheria

Q39. Complications of ANUG:

Ans. Gangrenous stomatitis or NOMA—caused by *Fusobacteium necrophorum.*

Q40. Difference between NUG and NUP:

Ans. NUP is when the advancing edge of NUG beyond the gingiva into the PDL space and into the bone.

Q41. Stress related lesions of oral cavity:

Ans. • Recurrent apthous stomatitis (RAS)
- Myofacial pain dysfunctional syndrome (MPDS)
- Acute necrotizing ulcerative gingivitis (ANUG)
- Recurrent herpes labialis (RHL)
- Burning mouth syndrome (BMS)
- Lichen planus (LP)

Q42. Treatment of ANUG:

Ans. • Amoxycillin
- Metronidazole
- Hydrogen peroxide (M/W)

Q43. Ulcers secondary to chemotherapy types:

Ans. Ulcers lack the erythematous halo
a. Direct (by methotrexate)
b. Indirect (bone marrow suppression by secondary to chemotherapy)

Q44. Ulcers without erythematous halo:

Ans. • Leukemia
- Cyclic neutropenia/Chédiak-Higashi syndrome
- Ulcers secondary to cancer chemotherapy

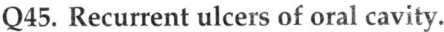

Q45. Recurrent ulcers of oral cavity.

Ans. • Recurrent apthous stomatitis (RAS)
• Recurrent EM
• Behçet's syndrome
• Recurrent HSV
• Recurrent ulcers in cyclic neutropenia

Q46. Etilogy of recurrent aphthous stomatitis.

Ans. • Immune mediated
• Haematologic
• Heredity
• Predisposing stress

Q47. Types of recurrent aphthous stomatitis (RAS)?

Ans. • Minor (Mikulicz disease)
• Major (Sutton's disease and PMNR—periadenitis mucosa necrotica recurrens)
• Herpetiform (Cook's apthae)

Q48. Difference between minor and major aphthous.

Ans. • Minor aphthae are a few mm and heals within 7–10 days without scarring
• Major aphthae lesions are >1 cm, more painful, heals in 10–30 day, with scarring

Q49. Syndromes associated with RAS recurrent aphthous stomatitis.

Ans. • PFAFA syndrome—periodic fever, aphthous, pharyngitis and adenitis.
• Behçet's syndrome
• Mouth and genital ulcers with inflamed cartilage (MAGIC).
• Sweet's syndrome

Q50. Characteristic features of aphthous ulcers.

Ans. • Starts as papule/ulcer
• No tissue tags
• Smooth, round, shallow, symmetrical

51. Differences between HSV and RAS.

HSV	RAS
Caused by HSV virus deficeincy	Caused by immunologic/nutritional
Begins as a vesicle and soon forms an ulcer	Begins as a papule/ulcer
SRSS ulcer with tissue tags	SRSS ulcer without tissue tags
Ulcers are in clusters	No cluster
Marginal gingivitis	No evidence of marginal gingivitis
Prodromal symptoms of fever, myalgia	Mild tingling before ulcer formation at that site
Cervical lymphadenopathy	No cervical lymphadenopathy
Treatment—topical antivirals, steroids contraindicated	Treatment—topical steroids
Tzanck cells seen	Anitschkow cells seen

Q52. Etiology of Behçet syndrome (silk route disease).

Ans. • Immune complexes
   • Recurrent oral/genital and eye lesions
   • Multisystem disorder—joints
      1. CVS
      2. CNS
      3. Renal
      4. Pulmonary disease

Q53. Diagnosis of Behçet's.

Ans. Pathergy test

Q54. What is the difference between recurrent ulcer and chronic ulcer.

Ans. Recurrent ulcers heal and form new ones in other site, whereas chronic ulcers are present at same site.

Q55. Etiology of pemphigus.

Ans. • Autoimmune related *acantholysis* leading to formation of *intraepithelial bullae.*

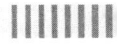

- Pemphigus can also be triggered by drugs like (3Ps and 1C) penicillin, penicillamine, phenylbutazone and captopril
- Pemphigus has been reported to coexist with other autoimmune diseases like (MTNL) myasthenia gravis, thymoma, non-Hodgkin lymphoma, chronic lymphocytic leukemia, Castleman disease and Waldenström's macroglobulinemia.

Q56. Classical signs in Pemphigus?

Ans.
- Nikolsky's sign which can be checked by application of lateral pressure on mucosa, by 3 way syringe and lifted with tweezer.
- Asboe-Hansen's sign—bulla enlarges by extension to an apparently normal surface.
- *Acantholysis* is the hallmark of pemphigus.

Q57. Types of pemphigus.

Ans.
- Pemphigus vulgaris
- Pemphigus vegetans
- Pemphigus erythematosus
- Pemphigus foliaceus
- Paraneoplastic pemphigus (PNPP) (associated with myasthenia gravis, thymoma, non-Hodgkin's lymphoma (MTNL)

Q58. Nikolsky's sign is positive in which conditions?

Ans.
- Pemphigus vulgaris
- Severe erythema multiforme
- Epidermolysis bullosa
- Ritter's disease (SSSS—staphylococcal scalded skin syndrome)

Q59. Etiology of pemphigoid.

Ans. Autoimmune related (subepithelial bullae salt-split skin)
- Bullous pemphigoid is also called ageing pemphigus and para pemphigus
- Mucous membrane pemphigoid also called ocular pemphigus and cicatricial pemphigoid

Q60. Oral lesions associated with eye involvement.

Ans. • Cicatrical pemphigoid (BMMP)

  • Reiter's syndrome

  • Behçet's syndrome

  • Stevens-Johnson syndrome

  • Hutchinson's triad in syphilis

  • Sjögren's syndrome

  • Herpes zoster

  • Hereditary benign intraepithelial dysplasia: HBID (seen as white lesions)

  • Hutchinson's triad in congenital syphilis.

Q61. Difference between pemphigus and pemphigoid.

Ans.

Pemphigoid	Pemphigus
Smaller lesions	Larger lesions
Form more slowly and bullae are intact for longer time	Bullae form early and rupture fast
Less painful	More painful
Less involvement present	Extensive labial involvement
Subepithelial bullae	Intraepithelial bullae

Q62. Ulcers causing scarring:

Ans. • Major aphthous

  • Ulcers of Behçet's disease

  • Ulcers of cicatricial pemphigoid

  • Epidermolysis bullosa

  • Lutic glossitis

  • OSMF

  • Burns

  • Multiple scelerosis.

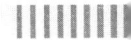

Q63. Ulcerative lesions in childhood?

Ans 1. Primary herpes simplex infections
   2. Riga-Fede's ulcers (associated with natal teeth in new borns)
   3. Mucocele

Q64. Ulcers associated with cervical lymphadenopathy.

Ans. 1. Primary herpes simplex infections
   2. ANUG
   3. Tuberculous ulcers
   4. Malignant ulcers
   5. Syphilitic ulcers.

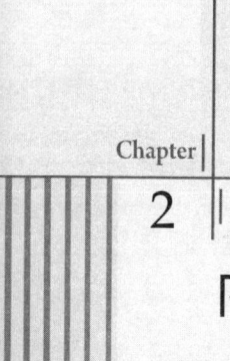

Red and White Lesions of Oral Cavity

Q1. Why are white lesions?

Ans.
- Increased keratinisation, e.g. leukoplakia, frictional keratosis.
- Increased thickening (acanthosis) of the epidermal covering (stratum spinosum) with
- increased production of keratin, e.g. lichen planus
- Coagulation of surface tissue (necrosis) such as it occurs in chemical/thermal burns.
- Formation of the pseudomembrane composed of desquamating epithelial cells, fibrin, inflammatory cells, micro-organisms and food debris, candidiasis
- Abnormal keratin production and imbibition of fluid (spongiosis) by the upper layers of the mucosa, e.g. leukoedema.

Q2. Mention scrapable and non-scrapable white lesions.

Ans. Scrapable:
- White coated tongue
- Thermal burns
- Chemical burns
- Sloughing traumatic lesion
- Diphtheria
- Acute pseudomembranous candidiasis

Non-scrapable

* Leukoplakia
* Lichen planus
* Nicotine stomatitis
* Leukoedema
* Linea alba
* Hyperplastic candidiasis
* Lupus erythematosus
* OSMF
* Actinic cheilitis

Q3. Mention the normal variants of oral mucosa which are white in color?

Ans. LFL—leukoedema, Fordyce's granules and linea alba

Q4. Mention nonkeratotic white lesions of oral cavity.

Ans. Nonkeratotic white lesions
  * Habitual cheek and lip biting
    – Burns
    – Uremic stomatitis
    – Radiation mucositis

Q5. In which infections white lesions are seen?

Ans. Bacterial
  * Syphilis
  * Diphtheria
  Viral
  * Hairy leukoplakia
  * Measles (Koplik's spots)
  Fungal
  * Candidiasis

Q6. Oral lesions with pseudomembrane formation.

Ans. * ANUG
  * Diphtheria
  * Uremic stomatitis

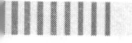

Q7. Mention red and white lesions with malignant potential.

Ans.
- Leukoplakia
- Erythroleukoplakia
- Carcinoma *in situ*
- Bowen's disease
- Oral submucus fibrosis
- Actinic keratoses, elastoses and cheilitis
- Discoid lupus erythematosus
- Dyskeratosis congenita
- Lichen planus

Q8. Define premalignant lesions and give some examples.

Ans. A **premalignant lesion** is a morphologically altered tissue in which cancer is more likely to occur than its apparently normal counterpart.
- Leukoplakia
- Erythroplakia
- Carcinoma *in situ*
- Actinic cheilitis
- Palatal changes associated with reverse smoking

Q9. Define premalignant conditions and give some examples.

Ans. A premalignant or precancerous condition is generalised state of the body in which cancer is more likely to occur.

Examples
- Lichen planus
- Syphilis
- Oral submucous fibrosis
- Plummer-Vinson syndrome (sideropenic dysphagia)
- Lupus erythematosus
- Dyskeratosis congenita

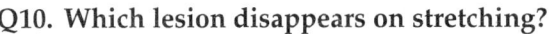

Q10. Which lesion disappears on stretching?

Ans. Leukodema
- *Velvet like veil* appearance
- Mother of pearl appearance

Q11. What are Fordyce granules?

Ans. Characterized by hyper tropic collection of sebaceous glands at various sites in the oral cavity. Appear as yellowish white spots.

Q12. What is Morsicatio buccarum?

Ans. Habits such as chronic lip, cheek or tongue chewing (Morsicatio buccarum/Linguarum)
Thickened shredded white areas with a irregular ragged/frayed surface.

Q13. Apperance of white lesions of burns.

Ans. May be caused by chemical, electrical or thermal means. Superficial pseudomembrane—necrotic surface tissue and inflammatory exudate.

Q14. What is uremic stomatitis?

Ans.
- Occurs in severe untreated renal failure (chronic) patients
- BUN levels >50 mg/dl
- Ulcers may be superficial or deep frequently involving the gingiva

Thickening of buccal mucosa which later includes a gray, thick, pasty, exudate and pseudomembrane covering the gingiva.

Q15. White lesions in syphilis.

Ans.
- Snail track ulcers
- Lutic glossitis (tufted tongue/upholstered tongue)—premalignant condition
- Other manifestations of syphilis
- *Primary:* Chancre formation
- *Secondary:* Mucus patches/Snail track ulcers/lutic glossitis
- *Tertiary:* Gumma and palatal perforation

Q16. Manifestations of congenital syphilis.

Ans.
- Frontal bossing
- Short maxilla
- High arched palate
- Saddle nose
- Hutchinson's teeth
- Higouménaki's sign
- Prognathic mandible
- Interatitial keratitis
- Rhagades
- Saber shin
- Eighth nerve deafness
- Scaphoid scapulae
- Clutton's joints

Hutchinson's triad –
- Hutchinson's teeth
- Ocular interstitial keratitis
- Eighth nerve deafness

Q17. What is the other name of candidiasis?

Ans. Thrush/moniliasis and candidosis or also known as disease of the diseased.

Q18. Classification of candidiasis

Ans. Acute
- Pseudomembranous (THRUSH)
- Atrophic (erythematous) (antibiotic stomatitis)

Chronic
- Atrophic: Denture sore mouth
  Angular cheilitis
  Median rhomboid glossitis
- Hypertrophic or hyperplastic
  - Candidal leukoplakia
  - Papillary hyperplasia of the palate
  - Median rhomboid glossitis (nodular)

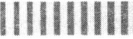

- Multifocal

Mucocutaneous: Syndrome associated, familial

Q19. Etiology of candidiasis.

Ans. *Candida albicans.* In HIV *Candida glabrata* and *Candida krusei* are also common

Q20. Predisposing factors of candidiais.

Ans.
- Premature infants/old age
  - Marked change in oral microbial flora: Excessive use of antibacterial mouth rinses, antibiotics
  - Xerostomia
  - Chronic local irritants (denture, ortho appliances)
  - Administration of corticosteroids (inhalational)
  - Poor oral hygiene/hospitalisation
  - Pregnancy and oral contraceptives
  - Immunologic deficiency (HIV, cancer chemotheraphy, radiotheraphy, leukaemia)
  - Malabsorption and malnutrition
  - Oral epithelial dysplasia.

Q21. What is secondary candidiasis?

Ans. It is oral manifestation of systemic mucocutaneous candidiasis (as a result of diseases such as thymic aplasia and candida endrocrinopathy syndrome)

Q22. What are the drugs that can cause candidiasis?

Ans. Corticosteroids (systemic and inhalational), cytotoxic drugs, immunosuppresants, radiation to head and neck. Marked changes in oral microbial flora may occur owing to administration of broad spectrum antibiotics, excessive use of mouth rinses, xerostomia secondary to anticholinergic agents or salivary gland diseases.

Q23. What is differential diagnosis of thrush?

Ans. Plaque form of lichen planus, leukoplakia, chemical burns

Q24. Types of denture sore mouth.

Ans. • *Type 1*: Pin point erythema
• *Type 2*: Diffused erythema
• *Type 3*: Palatal papillary hyperplasia (over riped strawberry appearance)

Q25. Etiology of angular chelitis.

Ans. Angular cheilitis is erythema, fissuring and scaling Involving the angles of the mouth. It is also called perleche, cheilocandidiasis. More common in diabetics

Etilogy
• Reduced vertical dimensions
• Nutritional deficiency
• Candida, co-infections with staphylococcus and β streptococci.

Q26. What are kissing lesions?

Ans. • Median rhomboid glossitis and chronic atrophic candidiasis on palate
• Chronic atrophic candidiasis on palate
• These lesions when they are combined are known as kissing lesions.

Q27. What is candidal leukoplakia?

Ans. Chronic hyperplastic candidiasis
• **Endogenous nitrosamine production; Candida acts as a co-carcinogen.**

Q28. What is ID reaction?

Ans. Allergic localised sterile vesiculopapular rash, also known as monolids.

Q29. Treatment of candidiasis?

Ans. • Elimination of predisposing factors
• Topical anti-fungal agents like
  – Nystatin 7–21 days of rinse 3–4 times daily. Cream form may be applied to the dentures and corner of the mouth.
  – Topical clotrimazole.

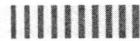

– Systemic anti-fungal agents
– Ketoconazole 200 mg once daily for 2 weeks
– Fluconazole 100 mg once daily for 2 weeks
– Itraconazole oral suspension 100–200 mg/day for
  2 weeks.

Q30. What is stomatitis nicotina palati. Is it premalignant?

Ans. A specific white lesion that develops on the palate of heavy cigarette, pipe and cigar smokers. The palatal mucosa becomes diffuse grey or white. Numerous slightly elevated papules with punctate red centers, it is not premalignant. Only oral changes associated with reverse smoking are premalignant.

Q31. What is geographic tongue?

Ans. Benign condition affecting primarily the dorsal surface of the tongue.
Also known as wandering rash of tongue and benign migratory glossitis and erythema circinata migrans.
Treatment: No treatment required.

Q32. What is dyskeratosis congenita?

Ans. White pigmented lesion associated with severely dystrophic nails, high incidence of oral cancer in young adults.

Q33. Etiology of white sponge nevus.

Ans. Due to a defect in normal keratinization of the mucosa, also known as Canon's disease. It is a hereditary condition.

Q34. EBV associated lesions?

Ans. • Oral hairy leukoplakia,
• Burkitt's lymphoma,
• Infectious mononucleosis, and
• Nasopharyngeal carcinoma.

Q35. Malignant potential of leukoplakia.

Ans. Type-wise : Homogenous **0.5–1.7%**
                    Speckled **20%**
       Site-wise : Floor of the mouth—**highest**

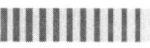

Q36. Etiology of leukoplakia.

Ans. Local

- Tobacco smokeless and smoking tobacco
- Alcohol
- Chronic irritation
- Candidiasis
- Electrogalvanic reaction

Systemic

- Syphilis
- Vitamin deficiency
- Sideropenic anameia (atrophy)
- Nutritional deficiency
- Xerostomia (loss of protective coating)
- Hormone
- Drugs
- Actinic radiation
- Virus (HSV, HPV 16 and 18)
- Idiopathic/cryptogenic

Q37. Clinical appearance of leukoplakia.

Ans. 'Cracked mud ' appearance,
Corrugated(ebbing tide), with a pattern of fine lines (cristae), wrinkled (dry-cracked mud) or papillomatous

Q38. Classification of leukoplakia.

Ans. Homogenous

- Flat
- Corrugated—ebbing tide appearance
- Pumice like (cristae)
- Wrinkled—cracked mud appearance

Non-homogenous

- Nodular or speckled
- Ulcerated and erythroleukoplakia

- Verrucous—oral florid papillomatosis
- Proliferative verrucous leukoplakia (PVL)

Q39. What is speckled leukoplakia?

Ans. It is non-homogenous type of leukoplakia. Due to combined appearance of white and red areas, the non-homogenous leukoplakia is also called erythro-leukoplakia and speckled leukoplakia

Q40. What is verrucous leukoplakia?

Ans. Verrucous leukoplakia is one in which the surface is broken up by multiple papillary projections that may also be heavily keratinized producing a lesion that bears some resemblance to the dorsum of the tongue.

Q41. What is proliferative verrucous leukoplakia?

Ans. Aggressive type of leukoplakia that almost invariably develops into malignancy.

Characterized by widespread and multifocal appearance, often in patients without known risk factors.

Q42. Differential diagnosis of leukoplakia.

Ans. Homogenous
  - Lichen planus
  - Leukoedema
  - Cheek biting lesion
  - Smokeless tobacco lesion
  - Discoid lupus erythematosus
  - Hyperplastic candidiasis
  - Hairy leukoplakia
  - Verrucous carcinoma
  - Verrucous vulgaris
  - White sponge nevus
  - Chemical burn
  - Syphilis
  - Psoriasis

Speckled
- Atrophic lichen planus
- Discoid lupus erythematosus

Q43. Investigations of leukoplakia.

Ans.
- Smear—to rule out candidal involvement
- Exfoliative cytology
- Toludine blue application
- Vizilite
- Velscope
- Histopathology
- Molecular analysis of DNA

Q44. What is toludine blue vital tissue staining?

Ans.
- Toludine blue (toludine chloride) is a metachromatic dye which stains mitochondrial DNA, cells with increase DNA and altered DNA in dysplastic or malignant cells.

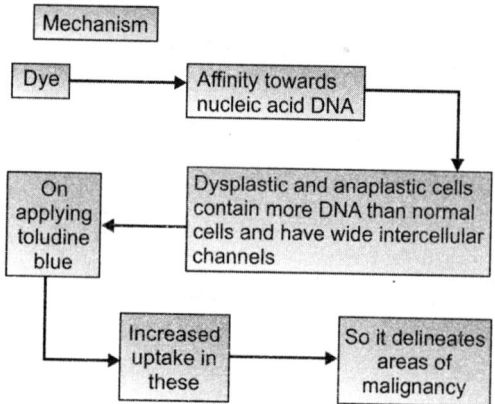

Indications
- Suspicious lesions
- Premalignant lesions
- To select the site for biopsy
- Mark the extent of the lesion for biopsy
- Postoperative evaluation—recurrence

Q45. Treatment of leukoplakia.

Ans. • Stop the habit

• Topical antifungal for 2 weeks

• Topical Vit A application—protective effect on the epithelium, antioxidant effect

Vit A 75000 to 300000 IU for 3 months

It may be used topically after painting with Beta carotene 5000 IU/day (chemo-prevention)—lycopene

• Topical bleomycin

• Cryosurgery

• Laser ablation

• Surgical stripping with graft coverage

• Excisional biopsy

Q46. Differential diagnosis of erythroplakia.

Ans. • Atrophic candidiasis

• Erosive lichen planus

• Lupus erythematosus

• Pemphigus

• Pemphigoid

• Tuberculosis

• Hemangioma

• Talangiectasia

• Kaposi's sarcoma

Q47. Etiology of oral lichen planus (OLP).

Ans. Cell-mediated immunity initiated by endogenous or exogenous factors.

Q48. Clinical features of OLP.

Ans. • Skin lesions have 6Ps: Purple, papular, pruritic, polygonal, platar and plaque like lesions

• Mean age 30–70 years

• Female predilection

- Wickham's striae, that produce either a lace like lesion or a pattern of fine radiating lines (linear) or annular lesions.
- Lesions are bi-lateral
- Koebner's phenomenon present.

Q49. Syndromes of OLP.

Ans. Grinspan syndrome-erosive OLP diabetes. Hypertension Graham Little syndrome—
  - Progressive patchy scarring. Hairloss of scalp.
  - Non-scarring thining of hair in armpits.
  - Spiky rough bumps on hair follicles.

Q50. Differential diagnosis of OLP.

Ans.
  - Leukoplakia
  - Candidiasis
  - Pemphigus
  - Lupus erythematosus
  - Drug induced
  - White sponge nevus
  - Ectopic geographic tongue
  - Cheek bite/frictional keratosis

Q51. What is malignant transformation rate of OLP?

Ans. Malignant transformation—0.5 – 2.5 %

Q52. Investigations of OLP.

Ans.
  - HB%, CT and BT liver function tests, HCV and FB
  - Biopsy
  - Immunofluoroscence—positive direct immunofluoroscence, at the level of basement membrane. Pattern may be globular or linear.

Q53. Treatment of oral lichen planus.

Ans.
  - Topical steroids
  - Triamcinolone acetate 0.01%
  - Clobetasol propionate

- Flucinonide
- Systemic steroids
- Prednisolone 20–40 mg early morning once a day (taper gradually)

Other modalities

- Topical cyclosporine rinses
- Systemic azathioprine
- Levamisole (immunomodulator)
- Dapsone (immunomodulator)
- Surgery (lasers, cryo)
- Photo-chemotherapy (PUVA)
- Vitamin A

Q54. What is the etiology of OSMF?

Ans. Areca quid chewing habit, vitamin deficiency and chillies.

Q55. Define OSMF?

Ans. An insidious chronic disease affecting any part of the oral cavity and sometimes the pharynx occasionally preceded

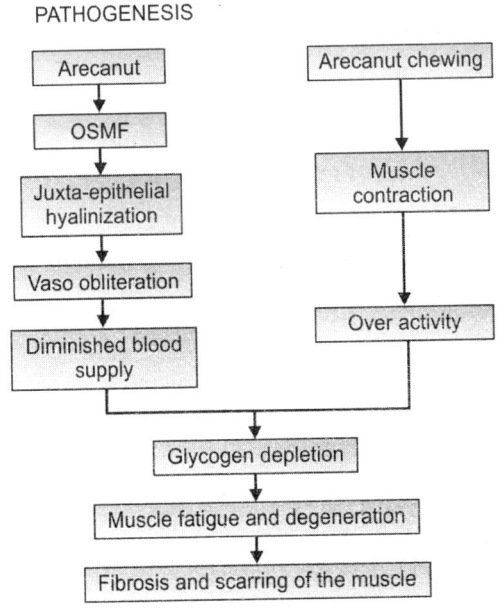

PATHOGENESIS

by and/or essociated with vesicle formation and always essociated with juxtaepithelial inflammatory reaction, followed by a fibroelastic change of lamina propria with epithelial atrophy leading to stiffness of oral mucosa and causing trismus and inability to eat.

Q56. Signs and symptoms of OSMF.

Ans. • Burning sensation of the oral cavity aggravated by spicy/hot food/fluids

• Vesiculation, excessive salivation, ulceration, pigmentation, recurrent stomatitis, defective gustatory sensations and dryness of mouth

• Gradual stiffening of oral mucosa after few years.

• Difficulty in swallowing when fibrosis extends to pharynx and esophagus

• Referred pain in ears, deafness and nasal voice

• Blanching, and Marble-like appearance to the oral mucosa

• *Soft palate:* Mobility is restricted when is involved.

• *Uvula: Shrunken bud* like or *hockey stick* appearance

Q57. Functional staging of OSMF

Ans. Stage 1: Mouth opening ≥20 mm

Stage 2: Mouth opening 11–19 mm

Stage 3: Mouth opening ≤10 mm

Q58. Treatment of OSMF.

Ans. • Elimination of the habit

• Nutritional support

• Bland diet

• Topical corticosteroids

• Physiotherapy

• Antioxidants

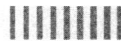

- Intralesional corticosteroids
- Intralesional corticosteroids with placentrix
- Intralesional corticosteroids with hyalurinadase
- Systemic—levamisole/dapsone
- Soft lasers
- Turmeric oil

Q59. Role of placentrix in OSMF?

Ans. • Accelerates cellular metabolism through HP axis
- Assisting in absorption of exudates—stimulation of regenerative process
- Increases physiological action of organs
- Anti-inflammatory, analgesic effects
- Increases blood circulation—tissue vascularity.

Q60. Role of hyaluronidase in OSMF.

Ans. Breaks down hyaluronic acid of the ground substance of the connective tissue and thereby causing increased penetration of steroids.

Q61. Which drugs are related to drug-induced lichenoid reaction?

Ans. Penicillin, gold, sulphonamides

Q62. Characterstic features of SLE.

Ans. Butterfly like rash on face and mixed red and white lesion seen in oral cavity.
Management is by topical steroids.

Q63. Geographic stomatitis features also seen in which other disease?

Ans. Reiter's disease or psoriasiform lesions.
Munro's microabscess associated with psoariasis.

Q64. Where is basket weave appearance seen?

Ans. White sponge nevus

Q65. What is malignant potential of various premalignant pathologies?

Ans. • **Leukoplakia**
- Homogenous leukoplakia—1–7%
- Verrucous leukoplakia—4–15%
- Speckled leukoplakia—18-47%
• Lichen planus—1–2%
• OSMF—3–6%

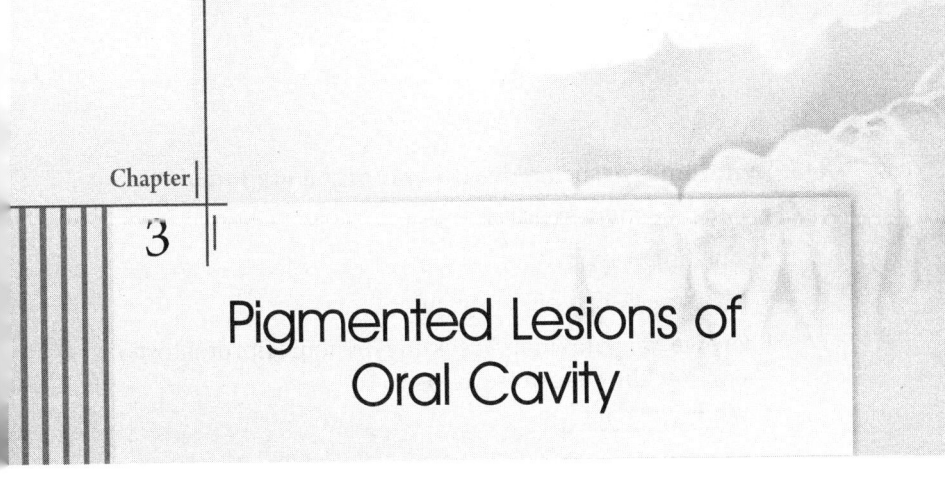

Pigmented Lesions of Oral Cavity

Q1. Name some common endogenous sources of mucosal color change.

Ans. Melanin, bilirubin, hemosiderin and hemoglobin.

Q2. Name the agents which are responsible for over-production of melanin?

Ans.   i. Increased sun exposure

ii. Physiologic source

iii. Neoplasia

iv. Medication or oral contraceptive use

v. High serum concentration of ACTH

vi. Postinflammatory changes

vii. Autoimmune/genetic

Q3. Which diagnostic tests are necessary for oral pigmentation?

Ans.   i. Diascopy

ii. Radiography

iii. Dermascopy/epiluminescence microscopy

iv. Blood test, e.g. serum ACTH

v. Binocular stereomicroscopes

vi. Use of hand held surfaces microscopes using incident light or oil immersion.

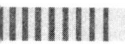

Q4. Syndromes associated with oral pigmentation.

Ans. • Peutz-Jeghers syndrome

• Cushing's syndrome

• McCune-Albright syndrome

• Crowe's sign (axillary freckling) in neurofibromatosis/ von Recklinghausans disease

• Addison's disease

• Laugier-Hunziker syndrome

• Sturge-Webers syndrome(red/blue)

• Rendu-Osler-Weber syndrome (hereditary Hemorrhagic telangiectasia) (red/blue)

Q5. Enumerate focal pigmented lesions.

Ans. • Amalgam tattoo (bluish gray macule adjacent to amalgam restoration)

• Oral melanotic macule

• Melanoma

• Pigmented nevus

• Melanoacanthoma

Q6. Enumerate multifocal/diffuse pigmented lesions.

Ans. • Physiologic pigmentation (especially in dark complexioned individual)

• Drug induced melanosis

• Smokers melanosis

• Inflammatory melanosis in oral lichen planus

• Peutz-Jeghers syndrome (intestinal polyposis) intraoral /perioral macules

• Laugier-Hunziker syndrome

• Addison's disease or Cushing syndrome

• Megaloblastic anemia

• Hyperthyroidism

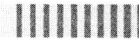

Q7. Define oral/labial melanotic macule and most common site involved in it.

Ans. Oral melanotic macule is benign pigmented lesion that has no known dermal counterpart.

Common sites: Lower lip and gingiva. Increased melanin production, no increase in melanocytes.

Q8. Conditions in which there is increased production of melanocytes?

Ans. • Melanocytic hyperplasia. This condition may have the potential of development of melanoma
• Melanocytic nevus
• Malignant melanoma.

Q9. Define melanocytic nevus and its types.

Ans. Increase in melanocytic growth and proliferation
Types:
    i. Intramucosal nevus
    ii. Common blue nevus
    iii. Compound nevus
    iv. Junctional nevus
    v. Combined nevus
    vi. Congenital nevus
    vii. Spitz nevus
    viii. Balloon cell nevus

Q10. Differentiate between nevus cell from native melanocyte.

Ans. • Nevi are immature form of melanocyte, ovoid, round and they have tendency to closely approximate one another.
• Melanocyte have dendritic morphology.

Q11. Syndromes associated with nevi.

Ans. • Turner's syndrome
• Noonan's syndrome
• Neurocutaneous melanosis.

Q12. Define junctional, compound and intramucosal nevi?

Ans. • When nevus cells are limited to the basal layer of epithelium, it is called junctional nevus.

• When nevus cells are in connective tissue, it is called intramucosal nevus.

• Nevus cells in basal region of epithelium and adjacent connective tissue is called compund nevus.

Q13. Which nevus has premalignant potential?

Ans. Blue nevus has a high rate of recurrence and has a high premalignant potential to become malignant melanoma.

ABCDE criteria to differentiate melanoma

A: Asymmetry

B: Irregular borders

C: Color variation

D: Diameter greater than 6 mm

E: Surface elevation.

Types

i. Superficial spreading melanoma

ii. Lentigo maligna

iii. Acral lentiginous

iv. Nodular melanoma

Superficial spreading melanoma. Lentigo maligna melanoma and acral lentiginous melanoma show radial growth phase and spread superficially and have a good prognosis.

Nodular melanoma shows a vertical growth phase with deeper invasion and have a poor prognosis, as there may be malignant melanoma formation.

Q14. Clinical apperance of oral melanoma.

Ans. Common site: Palate

Clinical feature: Macular, plaque like or mass forming circumscribed or irregular and exhibit focal or diffuse area of brown-blue or black pigmentation.

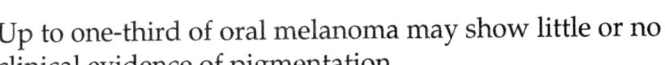

Up to one-third of oral melanoma may show little or no clinical evidence of pigmentation.

Q15. Define physiologic pigmentation and its differential diagnosis.

Ans. Physiologic pigmentation is of diffuse mucosal pigmentation in the childhood and does not develop denovo in adult.
Differential diagnosis
  i. Idiopathic
 ii. Drug induced
iii. Smoking induced melanosis
 iv. Endocrinopathic.

Q16. Drugs involved in drug-induced melanosis.

Ans. • Anti-malarial, e.g. chloroquine, hydroxychloroquine, quinacrine (as in treatment of LE).
• Phenothiazines, e.g. phenothiazines
• Oral contraceptive
• Cytotoxic medication, e.g. busulfan and cyclophosphamide.

Q17. Define melasma and chloasma.

Ans. • Melasma is generalized symmetric facial hyperpigmentation especially in females in reproductive years. It is called chloasma, if pigmentation occurs during pregnancy or with use of oral contraceptives.
• Treatment: Cessation of exogenous hormones
• It may spontaneously resolve after parturition.
• Topical administration of: 4%hydroquinone, 0.05% tretinoin and 0.01% fluocinolone acetonide
• And photoprotection with SPF 30 sunscreen.

Q18. Hormone disorder associated with pigmentation.

Ans. • Hypoadrenocorticism—generalized bronzing of the skin.
• Cushing's disease—moon facies, female predilection, weight gain.
• Hyperthyroidism

Q19. Diagnostic test for Addison's disease and Cushing syndrome.

Ans. • Addison's disease: Serum cortisol levels less than 100 nmol/L at 9.00 am
  • Hyponatremia
  • Hyperkalemia
  • Cushing syndrome:
      i. Low dose dexamethasone suppression test
      ii. Midnight plasma cortisol
      iii. 24 hr urinary free cortisol.

Q20. Clinical manifestation of primary biliary cirrhosis associated with pigmentation.

Ans. Diffuse mucocutaneous hyperpigmentation jaundice

Q21. Clinical feature of vitamin B$_{12}$ deficiency.

Ans. Megaloblastic anemia
  Generalized burning sensation, erythema and atrophy of mucosal tissue.

Q22. Describe Peutz-Jegher syndrome.

Ans. Hereditary intestinal polyposis, oral and perioral macular pigmentation.

Q23. What are café au lait spot and syndrome associated with it?

Ans. • Pigmentation resembling coffee in milk
  • Syndromes: Neurofibromatosis type 1 (Crowe sign-axillary freckling)
  • McCune Albright syndrome
  • Noonan's syndrome
  • The borders of pigmented lesion are described as
  • Jagged borders in McCune Albright syndrome resembling the Coast of Maine
  • Well defined borders in neurofibromatosis resembling Coast of California.

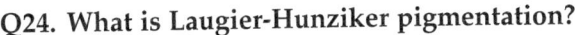

Q24. What is Laugier-Hunziker pigmentation?

Ans. • Seen in Caucasian or light skinned individuals

• Macules are not less than 5 mm in diameter on lips, buccal mucosa. Also esophageal, genital, and conjuctival mucosa, acral surfaces and nail involvement.

• Increased melanin pigmentation in basal cell layer without an increase in number of melanocytes and melanin incontinentia in superficial lamina propria.

• Differential diagnosis: Physiologic, drug or heavy metal induced pigmentation.

• Endocrinopathic disease

• Peutz-Jegher syndrome.

Q25. Write treatment plan for mucocutaneous and melanosis.

Ans. • Lasers CO_2, Nd: YAG and Q-switched alexandrite lasers.

• Fluocinolone combination of 4% hydroquinone, 0.05% retinoic acid, 0.01% acetonide.

Q26. Write about vitiligo.

Ans. • Etiology: Autoimmunity

• Cytotoxicity

• Genetics and alterations from metabolic and oxidative stress

• A single nucleotide polymorphism in vitiligo susceptibility gene associated with DM type 1, SLE, lupus erythematous and rheumatoid arthritis.

• Age group: Two-thirds decade of life.

• Pathology: There is destruction of melanocyte by antigen specific T cell and complete loss of melanin pigmentation

Treatment

– Topical corticosteriods

– Topical calcineurin inhibitors

- UVB narrow band
- Psoralen
- UVA exposure

Q27. Write etiology of petechiae and purpura.

Ans. • Amyloidosis
- Aplastic anemia
- Bulimia
- Chronic renal failure
- Forceful coughing

Q28. Causes of ecchymosis in oral cavity.

Ans. • Lesion due to trauma
- Leukemia
- End stage renal disease
- Bleeding and clotting disorders

Q29. How to differentiate ecchymosis/hematoma from port-wine stains?

Ans. Hematoma will be intially red and then turn brown in few days.

Q30. Etiology and complication of hemchromatosis.

Ans. • Etiology: Idiopathic
- Neonatal
- Blood transfusion
- Complication: Liver cirrhosis
- Bronzing of skin
- Diabetes
- Anemia
- Heart failure

Q31. Clinical features and management of amalgam tattoo.

Ans. Small, asymptomatic macular and bluish grey or even black in appearance. Can occur on gingiva, alveolar mucosa, buccal mucosa and floor of mouth.

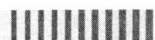

Q32. Clinical manifestation of graphite tattoo.

Ans. • Commonly seen on palate and gingiva

• It presents as solitary gray or black macule.

• Often occurs in childhood.

Q33. Heavy metal pigmentation.

Ans. • Silver cause generalized blue gray discoloration **(argyria)**

• Gold induce pigment may appear blue grey or purple **(chrysiasis)**

• Zinc oxide

Q34. Etiology and clinical manifestation of heavy metal pigmentation.

Ans. • Paints, old plumbing, sea food, industries.

• Grey to black appearance along free marginal gingiva

• Behavioral changes, neurological disorders

• Intestinal pain and sialorrhea.

Q35. Etiology of hairy tongue.

Ans. • Predisposing factor: Neglected oral hygiene

• Shift in oral microflora

• Antibiotics

• Immunosuppressive drugs

• Oral candidiasis

• Excessive alchol consumption

• Therapeutic radiation

• Black hairy tongue is associated with:

– Smoking tobacco

– Crack cocaine

• Use of psychotropic medication

• Tetracycline

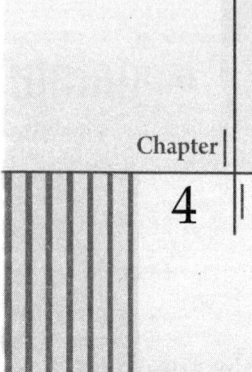

Oral Cancer

Q1. Differences between benign and malignant tumours.

Ans.

	Benign tumour	Malignant tumour
Metastasis	Absent	Present
Growth rate	Slow	Rapid
Ability to invade locally	Absent	Present
Recurrence rate	Low	High
Cellular appearance	Non-dysplastic	Dysplastic
Vascularity	Mild	Moderate to marked
Capsule	Present	Absent
Necrosis and ulceration	Absent	Present
Margins	Well defined	Infilterative and irregular
Effects on surrounding structures	Compresses the surrounding tissue	Invades and destroys surrounding tissue
Internal structure	Radiopaque- radiol ucent/mixed	Mostly radiolucent exception osteosarcoma
Effects on teeth	Displacement and smooth resorption	Resorption is rare. If present then spiked root resorption. Floating teeth appearance.
Treatment	Remove surgically	Surgery chemotherapy and radiotherapy

Q2. Define and enlist premalignant lesion and premalignant condition.

Ans. Premalignant lesion—a *morphologically altered* tissue in which cancer is more likely to develop than its apparently normal counterpart.

Examples:

- Leukoplakia
- Erythroplakia
- Palatal changes associated with reverse smoking
- Carcinoma *in situ*
- Bowen's disease
- Actinic keratosis, chelitis and elastosis kindly give space between headings of premalignant lesion and condition

Premalignant condition—*Generalised* state of body associated with increased risk of cancer.

Examples:

- OSMF
- Syphilis
- Oral lichen planus
- DLE
- Epidermolysis bullosa
- Sideropenic dysphagia (Plummer Vinson syndrome)
- Xeroderma pigmentosum

Q3. Etiology of oral cancer.

Ans. • Smoking
- Snuff and other forms of smokeless tobacco
- Betel and quid chewing
- Chronic irritation
- Sunlight—UV radiation
- Viruses
- Genetics

Q4. Clinical features of oral cancer.

Ans. • An ulcer in the mouth that does not heal
- A white or red patch
- A lump or thickening in the cheek
- A sore throat or a feeling that something is caught in the throat
- Difficulty chewing or swallowing
- Difficulty moving the jaw or tongue
- Presence of induration around the ulcer
- Proliferative lesion may be present
- Numbness of the tongue or other areas of the mouth
- Swelling of the jaw that causes dentures to fit poorly or become uncomfortable
- Loosening of the teeth or pain around the teeth or jaw
- Voice changes
- A lump or mass in the neck
- Weight loss
- The 6Ss involved in oral cancer are spirit, smoking, sunlight, syphilis, sharp tooth and sanguinara.

Q5. The common site for development of oral cancer in nonsmokers is:

Ans. Tongue

Q6. The common site for development of oral cancer in smokers is:

Ans. Floor of mouth

Q7. Plummer-Vinson syndrome is found to be associated with head and neck cancer of which region?

Ans. Post-cricoid region of hypopharynx

Q8. If pain occurs before swelling in a lesion, it is indicative of:

Ans. Inflammatory lesion, but if swelling occurs before pain in a lesion it is indicative of benign or malignant tumor.

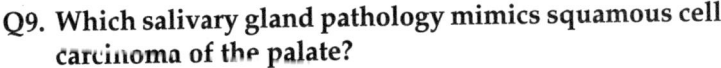

Q9. Which salivary gland pathology mimics squamous cell carcinoma of the palate?

Ans. Necrotizing sialometaplasia.

Q10. Features of oral cancer originating in maxillary sinus.

Ans. • If medial wall of sinus is involved = nasal obstruction may result.
- If superior wall of the sinus/floor of orbit is involved= displacement of the eye
- If lateral wall of the sinus is involved= bulging of the cheek
- If floor of the sinus/Roof of the oral cavity= growth in the palate

Q11. Which nodes are involved in oral carcinoma?

Ans. Submandibular, digastric and upper cervical nodes become hard and stony.

Q12. Enumerate the diagnostic aids for oral carcinoma?

Ans. • Toluidine blue staining
- Lugol's iodine
- Exfoliative cytology
- Oral CDx brush biopsy
- Chemiluminiscence
- Tissue fluoroscence imaging(ViziLite)
- Velscope
- Biopsy
- CT and MRI

Q13. Principle of toludine blue or vital tissue staining.

Ans. Toludine blue (toludine chloride) is a metachromatic dye which stains mitochondrial DNA, cells with increase DNA and altered DNA in dysplastic or malignant cells.

Q14. What is carcinoma *in situ*?

Ans. When dysplasia involves the entire thickness of the epithelium, it is known as carcinoma *in situ*.

Q15. Advantages for surgery as treatment modality for oral carcinoma.

Ans. • For tumors involving bone,
- • When the side effects of surgery are expected to be less significant than those associated with radiation
- • For tumors that lack sensitivity to radiation
- • For recurrent tumor in areas that have previously received radiotherapy.
- • Surgery also may be used in palliative cases to reduce the bulk of the tumor and to promote drainage from a blocked cavity.

Q16. Advantages of radiotherapy.

Ans. Radiation therapy has the advantage of treating the disease *in situ* and avoiding the need for the removal of tissue, and it may be the treatment of choice for many T_1 and T_2 tumors.

Q17. Which tumors are treated with external beam radiotherapy?

Ans. • Primary tumors of the posterior third of the tongue, oropharynx, and tonsillar pillar are best treated by external beam radiotherapy.
- • Custom Shells are commonly used for immobilisation and positioning of patients in radiotheraphy.

Q18. What is Brachytherapy?

Ans. In this interstitial and intracavitary implants may be used to treat primary tumors in head and neck region. Cesium, iridium and gold are isotopes used in brachytherapy.

Q19. What are the four 4Rs in fractionation?

Ans. Repair, reoxygenation, repopulation, redistribution

Q20. Side effects of chemotherapy.

Ans. Mucositis, nausea, vomiting, bone marrow suppression

Q21. Which sites in the oral cavity are associated with poorer prognosis?

Ans. Posterior aspect of oral cavity and oropharynx.

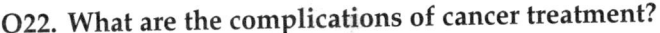

Q22. What are the complications of cancer treatment?

Ans.
- Mucositis,
- Hyposalivation,
- Candidiasis,
- Radiation caries,
- Tissue necrosis,
- Speech and mastication,
- Nutrition: Taste and smell impairment,
- Mandibular dysfunction, and
- Dentofacial abnormalities and pain

Q23. Metastatic tumors are most common in which region of the jaw?

Ans. Posterior mandible and maxilla.

Q24. Which sites in the jaw are most commonly involved presenting as secondary malignancy site?

Ans. Posterior areas of the mandible > maxillary sinus >Anterior hard palate > mandibular condyle.

Q25. Which malignant tumor is associated with bone deposition than resorption?

Ans. Osteosarcoma

Q26. What is malignant ameloblastoma and ameloblastic carcinoma

Ans. Malignant ameloblastoma is defined as an ameloblastoma with typical benign histologic features that is deemed malignant because of its biologic behavior, namely metastasis.
Ameloblastic carcinoma is an ameloblastoma exhibiting the histologic criteria of a malignant neoplasm such as increased and abnormal mitosis and large hyperchromatic, pleomorphic nuclei.

Q27. Which are the most common malignant tumors with matastasis in jaws?

Ans. Breast, kidney, lung, colon and rectum, prostate, thyroid, stomach, melanoma, testes, bladder, ovary, and cervix.

In children the tumors include neuroblastoma, retinoblastoma, and Wilms' tumor.

Q28. Which two bone lesions are known to convert into osteosarcoma osteosarcoma?

Ans. Fibrous dysplasia and Paget's disease

Q29. Characteristic features of multiple myeloma.

Ans.
- Also called myeloma, plasma cell myeloma, plasmacytoma
- It is the most common malignancy of bone in adults?
- **Bence Jones proteins** are seen in this lesion which results in foamy urine.
- Its radiographic features are **punched out radiolucency** (well defined without corticated borders).
- In this malignancy teeth appear too opaque/stand out conspicuously from their osteopenic background.

Q30. Characteristic features of non-Hodgkin's lymphoma.

Ans. Also called malignant lymphoma, lymphosarcoma
Extranodal sites in lymphoma are bone, skin, gastrointestinal mucosa, tonsils and Waldeyer's ring.

Q31. Features of Burkitt's lymphoma.

Ans. Other name African jaw lymphoma. Tumor doubling time is < 24 hrs and is hallmark of this tumor. This tumor show balloon like expansion

Q32. What are chloromas?

Ans. Foci of leukemic cells may be present as a mass that may behave like a localized malignant tumor.

Salivary Gland Disorders

Q1. Name the duct and site of orifice of salivary glands.

Ans. • Parotid (Stensons duct): Opening at buccal mucosa adjacent to maxillary 1st and 2nd molars
- Submandibular gland: Whartons duct opening at sublingual caruncle on either side of lingual frenum
- Sublingual gland (Bartholin's duct): Opening into submandibular duct.

Q2. Causes of xerostomia.

Ans. **i. Salivary causes**
- *Developmental:* Aplasia/Agenesis of gland/ Congenital stenosis of ducts
- *Autoimmune disease:* Sjogrens syndrome and Mickulicz disease

ii. Non-salivary causes
- Dehydration
- Irradiation
- Heerfordt's syndrome
- Anorexia bullosa nervosa
- HIV infected patient
- Drugs: TCAs, anticholinergic, antihypertensives
- Oral sensory disturbances
- Psychological disorders

Q3. What is Stafne's cyst?

Ans. It is a developmental salivary gland depression. Can be confirmed by sialography and CT. It is a psuedo-cyst.

- Stafne's cyst presents between angle of mandible and first molar below the level of inferior alveolar canal
- Usually asymptomatic and appears on radiograph as a round, unilocular, well circumscribed radiolucency.
- Can be present both anteriorly and posteriorly.

Q4. Which gland is more affected in sialolithiasis and why?

Ans. More common in submandibular gland because of tortuous course of duct, comma-shaped anatomy of duct (right angle bend), higher calcium and phosphate levels and dependent position of submandibular gland.

Q5. Indications of sialography.

Ans. • To detect calculus/sialolith
- To determine the extent of destruction of gland due to obstruction
- To detect fistulae and diverticuli in salivary glands
- To detect and diagnose recurrent swellings and inflammatory process
- To detect site, size and origin of tumor
- To outline the plane of facial nerve as guide for biopsy or dissection

Q6. Contraindications of sialography.

Ans. • Acute infections.
- May interfere in thyroid function tests.
- Allergy to iodine.

Q7. Differences between oil-based and water-based contrast media.

Ans.

Oil-based contrast media	Water-based contrast media
Viscous in consistency	Low viscosity
Pressure induction needed	Rapid and easy induction
Slow removal	Rapid removal
Good contrast	Decreased contrast

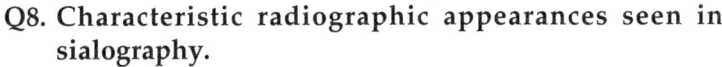

Q8. Characteristic radiographic appearances seen in sialography.

Ans. • Normally, leafless tree appearance is seen
  – *Bush in winter* appearance in submandibular gland
  – *Tree in winter* appearance in parotid
• Radiolucent voids, known as "filling defect" are seen in radiolucent sialoliths
• *Cherry blossom* appearance in Sjögren's syndrome (salt and pepper appearance on MRI)
• *Sausage string* appearance: Sialodochitis
• *Ball in hand* appearance in benign tumours
• Puddling of contrast agent in malignant tumours

Q9. Applications of saliva as a diagnostic aid.

Ans. • To determine viral infections
• Alcohol consumption
• Assess hormone levels
• Screening for cancers and other systemic diseases

Q10. Imaging/radiographic views for salivary gland disorders.

Ans. • Panaromic
• Lateral oblique
• Anteroposterior (AP)
• Puffed cheek AP
• Occlusal, to see sialolith in the Wharton's duct
• OPG to see sialolith in the gland

Q11. Clinical features of xerostomia.

Ans. Signs
• *Lipstick* sign
• *Tongue blade* sign
• *Schirmer's test* (paper strip inserted in eye to measure the tears—less than 5 mm in 5 minutes in Sjögren's syndrome)

- BUT (break up time test—time for ocular surface to lose cohesiveness after each blink),
- Rose Bengal dye test to stain damaged corneal cells
- Scintigraphy
- Sialography
- MRI—salt and pepper appearance in Sjögren's syndrome
- Salivary flow rates,
- Serology,
- Cytology,
- Minor salivary gland biopsy: Labial glands: Most confirmatory
- DMFT scores

Symptoms
- Postmenopausal females
- Bilateral enlargement of parotid glands
- Lips are cracked, peeling, atrophic
- Tongue is smooth, reddened with loss of papillation
- *Caries decay on root surfaces and cusp tip involvement*
- Debris accumulation in interproximal regions
- Periodontal pathology
- Candidiasis
- Angular cheilitis
- Saliva is viscous and scant secretions
- Hazy flocculated accretions and clumped epithelial cells which lend the saliva a cloudy appearance
- Enlarged and painful gland is indicative of acute inflammation
- Facial nerve paralysis

Complications of Sjögren's syndrome: Lymphoma

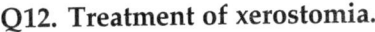

Q12. Treatment of xerostomia.

Ans. • Preventive therapy: Supplemental fluorides, remineralising solutions, optimal oral hygiene and diet, antifungal.

• Symptomatic treatment: Methyl cellulose, artificial saliva and tears, oral rinses, mouthwashes, increased humidifiers, aloevera gel.

• Local or topical stimulation: Sugar free gums and mints, acupuncture, electric stimulation.

• Systemic stimulation: Secretogogues like cevimeline (30 mg tds), pilocarpine, bromohexine, anetholehithione.

• Therapy of underlying systemic disorders: Anti-inflammatory therapy.

Q13. Characteristic sites for salivary gland disorders.

Ans. • Bacterial sialadenitis: Parotid gland(because of ascending infection and the mucin content in parotid is comparatively less than submandibular gland leading to increased chances of infection, decreased bacteriostatic activity and resting flow levels).

• Ranula (retentive mucocele): Sublingual gland floor of mouth

• Mucocele: Extravasation mucocele on lower lip

• Mumps: Parotid gland

• Sialolith: Submandibular gland (because of tortuous course of duct, comma shaped anatomy of duct, higher calcium and phosphate levels, dependent position of submandibular gland)

• Mucoepidermoid carcinoma: Parotid gland (major salivary gland)

Palate (minor salivary gland)

• Adenoid cystic carcinoma: Submandibular gland (ACC is having perineural invasion).

Q14. Which gland is mostly affected in Sjögren's syndrome?

Ans. • Parotid gland.

15. **What are the confirmatory tests for Sjögren's syndrome?**

Ans. Minor salivary gland biopsy:
   - Number of infiltrating mononuclear cells, aggregate of 50 or more cells is called a focus
   - Number of foci per 4 mm is calculated (focus score of >1 is positive)
   • Presence of autoantibodies against anti-SS-A(Ro) and anti-SS-B(La)
   • Ocular examination: Rose Bengal dye, Schirmer's test

Q16. **Differential diagnosis of salivary gland swelling.**

Ans. • Unilateral:
   - Pleomorphic adenoma
   - Sialoadenitis
   - Mumps
   • Bilateral:
   - Mickulicz disease
   - Mumps
   • Warthin's tumor
   • CMV mononucleosis
   • Sialosis
   • Bacteremia
   • Bulimia
   • Diabetes mellitus
   • Alcohol
   • Oncocytoma
   • Sarcoidosis
   • HIV-associated benign lymphoepithelial hypertrophy.

Q17. **Classification of Sjögren syndrome.**

Ans. • Primary Sjögren: Xerostomia, xerophthalmia,
   • Secondary Sjögren: Xerostomia, xerophthalmia, and underlying autoimmune disease such as SLE, RA or scleroderma.

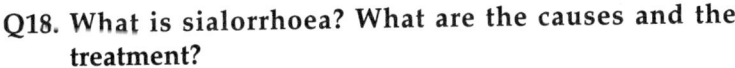

Q18. What is sialorrhoea? What are the causes and the treatment?

Ans. • Excessive secretion of saliva or hypersalivation.

Causes
- Medications: Pilocarpine
- Cevimiline
- Lithium
- Bethanechol
- Physostigmine
- Clozapine
- Risperidone
- Nitrazepam
- Neurologic disease: Parkinson disease, Wilson' s disease, amyotrophic lateral sclerosis, Down syndrome, Fragile X syndrome, autism, cerebral palsy.
- Heavy metals: Iron, lead, arsenic, mercury, thallium.

Treatment
- Physical therapy: Speech and swallowing therapy to improve neuromuscular control.
- Medications: Compatible xerostomic agents –
- Scopolamine
- Transdermal agents
- Propantheline
- Benztropine
- Glycopyrrolate
- Diphenhydramine
- Hydrochloride
- Surgery: Duct ligation or excision of one or more salivary gland.

Q19. Different necrotic lesions of oral cavity.

Ans. • Necrotising sialometaplasia
- Acute necrotizing ulcerative gingivitis

- Necrotizing ulcerative periodontitis
- Noma or gangrenous stomatitis

Q20. Radiation dose that can cause permanent damage to the salivary glands?

Ans. More than 24–26 Gray

Q21. What is Mumps?

Ans.
- Caused by paramyxovirus (RNA)
- Transmitted by direct contact with salivary droplets.
- Contagious
- Especially in children associated with fever and bilateral painful swelling of parotid gland.

Q22. Complications of mumps:

Ans.
- Encephalitis
- Meningitis
- Oophoritis
- Testicular atrophy
- Infertility
- Deafness
- Myocarditis
- Orchitis

Q23. Role of scintigraphy in salivary gland disorders.

Ans.
- Provides quantitative information on the functional capabilities of the gland
- Used to aid in diagnosis of ductal obstruction, sialolithiasis, Gland aplasia, bell's palsy, Sjögrens syndrome

Q24. What are phases of sialography?

Ans.
- Flow phase: 15–20 sec
- Concentration phase: 1 min after administration
  - After 10 min it increases in gland
  - After 15 min it increases in oral cavity and decreases in gland
- Washout phase: Application of lime/citric acid after 1 hr

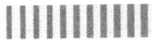

Q25. Characteristic appearances on scintigrapy of salivary gland disorders.

Ans. • Hot spot—acute inflammation, oncocytoma, Warthin's tumor

• Cold spot—Sjögren syndrome, rest of the salivary tumors (malignant tumors seen as cold spot with fuzzy margins and benign tumors are seen as cold spot with regular margins)

• Panda eye appearance in sarcoidosis.

Q26. Etiology of sialoliths.

Ans. Inflammation, irregularities in ductal system, local irritants and anticholinergic medication lead to pooling of saliva.

Q27. Complications of sialolith formation.

Ans. • Pain just before eating

• Enlarged and tender–gland

• Decreased/stasis of saliva may lead to infection, fibrosis and atrophy

• Fistula or sinus formation over the stone.

Q28. Treatment of sialolith.

Ans. • Stones on the surface are removed from duct by milking of gland

• Deeper stones require removal using surgery or sialoendoscopy

• Lithotripsy (effective for parotid than submandibular gland)

Q29. Describe mucocele.

Ans. • Accumulation of saliva at the site of traumatized or obstructed minor salivary gland duct. Occurs unilaterally. Common site: Lower lip, it is a pseudocyst and mucus extravasation type of cyst

• Differential diagnosis: Dermoid cyst

Q30. Describe ranula.

Ans. • Resembles abdomen of frog
  • Usually lesions occur on one side of lingual frenum but it can occur bilaterally if deep
  • A deep lesion that herniates through the mylohyoid muscle and extends along the facial planes is known as *plunging ranula*
  • Radio-opaque material instilled in the ranula may be helpful in delineating the borders and full extent of the lesion.

Q31. What precautions during radiotherapy can reduce xerostomia?

Ans. • Improvement in planning and delivery of radiotherapy.
  • **Radioprotective agents** may help limit radiation therapy **(amifostine)**
  • Amifostine is administered intravenously or subcutaneously 15–30 min prior to each fractionated radiation therapy.
  • Mechanism of action involves the intracellular scavenging of free oxygen radicals.

Chapter

6

Temporomandibular Joint Disorders

Q1. How is TMJ unique from other joints of the body?

Ans. Distinguishing features of TMJ are:
1. Fibrocartilage is present instead of hyaline cartilage
2. Avascular tissue is present named as retrodiscal tissue
3. Ginglymoarthrodial type of joint simultaneous, coordinated movements

   Hinge + Gliding movements

Q2. Ligaments associated with TMJ.

Ans. 1. Capsular ligament
2. Lateral temporomandibular ligament
3. Stylomandibular ligament
4. Sphenomandibular ligament

Q3. Muscles of mastication.

Muscle	Origin	Insertion	Function
Masseter	From maxillary process of zygomatic bone. Superficial part of maxillary process of zygomatic bone and the anterior two-thirds of the inferior part	Lateral aspect of ramus	Together forms a sling and produces powerful forces of chewing

(Contd.)

61

(Contd.)

Muscle	Origin	Insertion	Function
Medial pterygoid	Medial surface of lateral ptery-goid plate	Medial aspect of ramus	Closing of mandible
Temporalis	Temporal fascia	Coronoid pro-cess and mandi-bular ramus.	Fan-shaped opening and Retrusion of mandible.
Lateral pterygoid	Inferior part: Lateral surface of lateral ptery-goid plate. Superior part: Greater wing of sphenoid	Anteromedial aspect of con-dylar neck and disc	Main protrusive and opening muscle
Digastric (accessory muscle)	Anterior belly from digastric fossa of mandible. Posterior belly from mastoid notch of temporal	Together they insert on the hyoid bone	Depression and retrusion of mandible
Buccinator accessory muscle)	From the alveolar processes of maxilla and man-dible, and ptery-gomandibular raphe	Orbicularis oris	Compresses cheek into the teeth for chewing

Q4. Etiology of TMJ disorders.

Ans. a. Instability of maxilllomandibular relationships.

b. TMJ hypermobility

c. Trauma(dental procedures, oral intubation for GA, yawning, microtrauma and macrotrauma)

d. Parafunctional activity (sleep bruxism, clenching, lip or cheek biting).

e. Sleep disturbance

f. Comorbidity, e.g. rheumatic/musculoskeletal or pain disorders/gouty arthritis

g. Emotional stress.

Q5. What is the normal range of motion or mouth opening?

Ans. 40–50 mm

Q6. Clinical diagnostic tests for TMJ.

Ans. a. Thermography

b. Jaw tracking

c. EMG

Q7. Treatment of myofacial pain.

Ans. 1. Educate to perform self care and reassurance

2. Controlled parafunctional activity

3. Physical therapy; heat and cold therapy, ultrasound, laser, TENS.
   – Passive stretching exercises
   – Trigger point therapy

4. Intraoral appliance therapy;repositioning splints

5. Pharmacotherapy; NSAIDs, Muscle relaxants, anti-anxiety agents, tricyclic antidepressants, capsaicin

6. Behavioral and relaxation therapy; hypnosis, biofeed-back, cognitive behavioural therapy.

Q8. Laskin's diagnostic criteria for TMJ.

Ans. 1. Facial pain in the region of TMJ

2. Limitation or deviation in mandibular movements.

3. Hyperalgesia of musculoskeletal structures.

4. TMJ sounds during jaw function and movement.

Q9. Types of articular disc displacement.

Ans. 1. Anterior disc displacement with reduction

2. Anterior disc displacement without reduction

Q10. Most common type of disc displacement is:

Ans. Anterior and medial to the condyle.

Q11. Management of anterior disc displacement.

Ans. a. Splint therapy
b. Physical therapy
c. Anti-inflammatory drugs
d. Arthrocentesis
e. Arthroscopic lysis and lavage
f. Arthroplasty
g. Vetical ramus osteotomy

Q12. Symptoms of septic arthritis.

Ans. Trismus, deviation of mandible to the affected side, severe pain on movement, inability to occlude the teeth, inflammation of the joint space, a large tender cervical lymph nodes. Sequelae of septic arthiritis—osteomyelitis of temporal bone, brain abscess, ankylosis.

Q13. What is difference between TMJ dislocation and subluxation?

Ans. In dislocation the condyle is positioned anterior to the articular eminence and cannot return to its normal position without assistance.
And in subluxation, condyle moves anterior to the eminence during wide opening anterior to the eminence during wide opening but is able to return to the resting position without manipulation.

Q14. Characteristic clinical sign of anterior dislocation.

Ans. Preauricular hollow in joint space.

Q15. Definition of ankylosis/stiff joint.

Ans. Pathological fusion of parts of joint resulting in restricting movement across the joint.
Types of ankylosis
a. Fibrous ankylosis
b. Bony ankylosis

Q16. Characteristic features in MPDS.

Ans. • Females more commonly affected.
• Trigger points exist as localized tender areas within taught bands of skeletal muscles and when stimulated

refers a characteristic pain pattern to a distant group of muscles.

- Palpation of trigger points will give rise to a positive 'jump sign'.
- No biochemical or radiographic findings in MPDS.

Q17. Difference between disc displacement with reduction and disc derangement with reduction:

Ans.

Disc displacement with reduction	Disc displacement without reduction
Opening and closing reciprocal click	Clicking absent
Pain on opening	Restricted mouth opening
	Closed lock <35–40 mm
Deviation to affected side	Deflection to affected side
Click on lateral excursion	Protrusive and lateral movements restricted

Q18. Syndromes associated with condylar hypoplasia:

Ans.
- Treacher Collins syndrome
- Pierre Robin's syndrome
- Mandibulofacial dysostosis
- Therapeutic radiation

Q19. Features of coronoid hyperplasia.

Ans. Difficulty in mouth opening, Best seen on Waters view

Q20. Define oral dyskinesia.

Ans. These are the abnormal involuntary movements of the tongue, lips and jaw.

Q21. Deviation of mandible is toward which side in anterior disc displacement without reduction?

Ans. Towards the side of click

Q22. In unilateral TMJ ankylosis chin is displaced towards which side?

Ans. Towards affected side.

Q23. **In unilateral condylar hypoplasia deviation of chin toward which side?**

Ans. On the involved side.

Q24. **In unilateral condylar hyperplasia deviation of chin toward which side?**

Ans. On the opposite side.

Q25. **In unilateral TMJ dislocation chin deviated to which side?**

Ans. Towards the opposite side.

Orofacial Pain

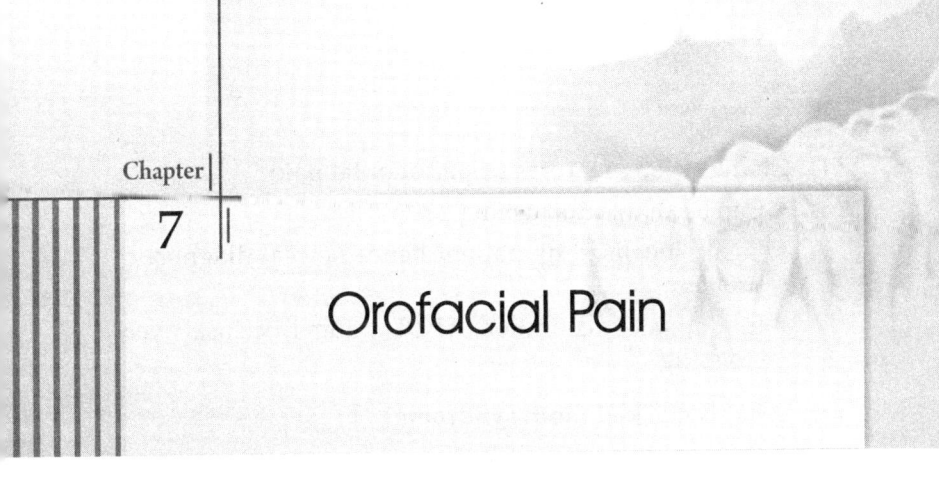

Q1. What is pain?

Ans. Definition of pain: IASP defines pain as an unpleasant sensory and emotional experience associated with actual or potential tissue damage or described in terms of such damage.

- A delta and C fibers are the principal nociceptors

A delta	1–6mm in diameter	Myelinated	5–30 m/s conduction velocity	First pain experienced–sharp
C delta	1.5 mm in diameter	Nonmye-lineted	0.5–2m/s conduction velocity	Steady dull pain

Q2. What is gate control theory?

Ans. Gate control theory: Larger fibers having higher conduction velocity reach the substantia gelatinosa of the spinal cord faster and block the gate resulting in inhibition or decreased sensitivity to impulses from the smaller fibers.

Q3. Characteristic features of pulpal pain.

Ans.
- Can be acute/chronic
- Difficult to localise by patient
- Presence of pathology—obvious/obscure
- Increased by heat and cold
- Nature varies over time. Sharp may become dull, e.g. rubbing at the site of pain decreases the pain stimulus

Q4. Characteristic features of periodontal pain.

Ans. • Can be sharp/dull aching
- Easily localised by patient hence no real diagnostic problem
- Inflammatory condition of PDL, trauma, occlusal over stressing

Q5. What is cracked tooth syndrome?

Ans. • Pain on biting and releasing biting pressure
- Pain in particular occlusal position
- Diagnosis
  - Rubber wheel test
  - Transillumination
  - Application of dye

Q6. What is Barodontalgia?

Ans. • Pain in tooth due to change in atmospheric pressure
- Summation of neural impulses is etiology
- For example, scuba divers and mountaineers

Q7. What are the characteristics of cardiac pain?

Ans. • Aching pain is cyclic
- Referred to left angle of mandible
- Associated with chest pain
- Worsens after exertion
- Relief with nitroglycerine

Q8. Types of neuralgic pain.

Ans. Types of neuralgia:
- Trigeminal
- Glossopharyngeal (pain in region of tonsil and ear)
- Geniculate
- Superior laryngeal
- Occipital

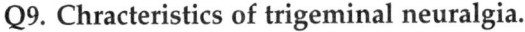

Q9. Chracteristics of trigeminal neuralgia.

Ans. Trigeminal neuralgia (tic douloureux)

Etiology

- Compression and demyelination of nerve root
- Causes ectopic firing of focal group of ganglion neurons
- For example, compression of trigeminal nerve by sup. cerebral artery,
- Compression by expanding cranial tumours
- Systemic multiple sclerosis

Clinical manifestations

- Most commonly observed neuralgia by dentists
- Sharp lancinating, electric shock like pain
- Lasts for a short time
- Trigger zones provoked by light touch
- Refractory periods seen
- Mostly unilateral
- Rapid bilateral involvement suggests multiple sclerosis

Q10. Treatment of trigeminal neuralgia.

Ans. Treatment

A. Medicinal

i. Carbamazepine:

Mode of action: Blocks Na channels, reduces potentiation in spinal cord, reduces synaptic transmission in trigeminal nucleus .

Dosage: 100 mg/day, initially then increased, maximum up to 800–1200 mg/day.

Side Effects

- Renal and hepatic toxicity
- Blurring of vision
- Unsteadiness
- Haematopoietic depression, causing aplastic anemia—regular blood counts are advised.

ii. Baclofen

- It is a muscle relaxant
- Less toxic and less efficacious than carbamazepine

    Dose: 10 mg/day, increased to 80 mg/day

    Side effects: Drowsiness and confusion

iii. Pimozide—more effective than carbamazepine, but more toxic.

iv. Gabapentin—increases GABA levels

    Dose: 300 mg on 1st day, 300 mg bid 2nd day, 300 mg tds from 3rd day no abrupt stoppage

v. Tocainide-haematologic toxicity observed

vi. Topical Capsaicin

Surgical

- Alcohol injection
- Injection of boiling water
- Neurectomy
- Gangliolysis
- Decompression
- Gamma knife
- Tractotomy
- Rhizotomy

Q11. What is Facial Palsy?

Ans. Facial Palsy (Bell's palsy)

- Due to inflammation of facial nerve within facial canal
- Causes facial paralysis and burning pain in auricular area
- Transitory facial paralysis results due to angioneurotic oedema, which subsides on control of angioneurotic oedema

Q12. Characteristic features of pain associated with herpes zoster.

Ans.
- **Unilateral** acute neuritis of viral source (varicella zoster)
- Prodromal symptoms of burning, followed by tiny vesicles, leaving cutaneous and mucosal ulcerations unilaterally.
- Difficult to diagnose in early stage of prodromal burning
- Superficial distribution according to anatomic pattern of nerve fibres
- After vesicle formation diagnosis is obvious
- Nerve block does not relieve pain, hence differentiated from trigeminal and glossopharyngeal neuralgia.

Q13. What is postherpetic neuralgia?

Ans.
- Chronic unilateral burning pain superficially in area affected by acute attack of HZ
- Pain accompanied by hyperalgesia of healed scar
- Due to re-activation of virus, latent in ganglion
- Previous H/o herpes zoster is diagnostic

Treatment
- Topical: Anesthetics, capsaicin, EMLA
- Systemic: Carbamazepine, phenytoin, gabapentin
Steroids are used but controversial

Q14. What is burning mouth syndrome?

Ans.
- Typical in older females
- Spontaneous onset
- Most common at anterior part of tongue, hard palate and lower lip
- Sleep is not disturbed
- Spontaneous remission in some cases

Etiology
- Menopause
- Nutritional factors

- Diabetes
- Neuropathy
- Mechanical trauma
- ACE inhibitors
- Sleep disorders

Q15. Differential diagnosis of burning mouth syndrome.

Ans.
- Odontogenic pain
  - Oral lichen planus
  - Candidiasis
  - Oral submucous fibrosis
  - Trigeminal neuralgia
  - Xerostomia
  - Maxillary sinusitis
  - TMJ pain
  - Postherpetic neuralgia

Q16. Treatment of burning mouth syndrome:

Ans.
- Low dose amitriptyline
  - 15–30 mg chlordiazepoxide
  - Clonazepam 0.5–6 mg.

Oral Manifestations of HIV

Q1. What is HIV virus?

Ans. It is human immunodeficiency virus

- It is a retrovirus.
- Characterized by reverse transcriptase activity which converts viral RNA to provirus DNA.
- RNA virus also called Lente virus/Retrovirus

Q2. Spread of HIV virus.

Ans.
- Sexual intercourse
- Mother to fetus (perinatal)
- Contaminated blood, blood products (parentral)

Q3. Signs and symptoms of HIV infection.

Ans. Characterized by immunosuppression, leads to spectrum of clinical manifestations that includes opportunistic infections, secondary neoplasms and neurologic manifestations.

Most common signs and symptoms:

- Fever
- Fatigue
- Maculopapular rash
- Headache
- Lymphadenopathy

Infections

Fungal

- Candidiasis
- Cryptococcosis
- Histoplasmosis
- Aspergillosis
- Mucormycosis

Viral

- Herpes simplex infection (RIOII and RHL—recurrent intraoral herpes infection and recurret herpes labialis)
- Human papillomavirus infection (papilloma and condyloma papilloma)
- Herpes zoster infection/virus (HZV)
- Epstein-Barr virus infection (oral hairy leukoplakia)
- Cytomegalovirus infection
- Pox virus (molluscum contagiosum)

Bacterial

- Linear gingival erythma (LGE)
- Necrotising ulcerative gingivitis and periodontitis (NUG and NUP)
- Syphilis
- Tuberculosis
- Bacillary angiomatosis
- Actinomycosis
- Cat-scratch disease

Neoplasm

- Kaposis-Sarcoma (HHV-8)
- Non-Hodgkin lymphoma

Immune mediated

- Major aphthous
- Non-specific ulceration—neutropenic ulceration

Miscellaneous/others

- Thrombocytopenia
- Xerostomia
- Parotid disease (sialosis)

Revised surveillance case definition for HIV infection

Stage	Lab evidence	Clinical evidence
Stage I	Lab confirmation of HIV infection and CD4 + T lymphocytes ≥ 500/µl	None required (but no AIDS defining condition)
Stage II	Lab confirmation of HIV infection and CD4 + T lymphocytes 200–499/µl	None required (but no AIDS defining condition)
Stage III	Lab confirmation of HIV infection and CD4 + T lymphocytes <200/µL	Documentation of AIDS defining condition (with lab confirmation of infection)

Q4. What are the stages in HIV infection?

Ans. 1. Acute primary infection/seroconversion

- Majority of HIV seroconversion are asymptomatic
- Small number of patients present with self-limiting non-specific illness characterized by fever, arthralgia, myalgia, lymphadenopathy
- Lab. findings—WBC decrease CD4 count decrease
- CD4 : CD8 ratio is reversed.

2. Asymptomatic infection

- Majority are asymptomatic, remains infectious due to continued replication of virus
- Duration of asymptomatic period is variable but mean of 10 years from infection to development of AIDS has been suggested
- Most commonly employed parameters include
  - Decrease in CD4 count
  - Increase in CD8 count
  - CD4:CD8 ratio reversed
  - Increased p24 antigen
  - Decreased p24 antibody

3. **Persistent generalised lymphadenopathy**
   - Patient with asymptomatic HIV infection presents with persistent generalised lymphadenopathy (> 1 cm of two or more extrainguinal sites for > than 3 months).

4. **Symptomatic HIV infection**
   - Susceptibility to opportunistic infection with tumor
   - Presence of multiple infection
   - Lack of typical sign and symptom due to failure of inflammatory response.

Q5. Classification of HIV.

Ans. **Revised CDC Classification of HIV (1993)**
   Group I lesion strongly associated with HIV
   - Candidiasis
     - Erythematous
     - Pseudomembranous
   - Hairy leukoplakia
   - Kaposi sarcoma
   - Non-Hodgkin lymphoma
   - Periodontal disease
     - Linear gingival erythema
     - NUG
     - NUP

   Group II lesion less commonly associated
   - Bacterial: *Myco. avium* intercellulare
     - *M. tuberculosis*
     - Necrotizing ulcerative stomatitis

   Group III lesion seen in HIV
   - Bacterial infection—*Actinomyces israelle*
     - *E. coli*
     - *K. pneumoniae*
     - Cat scratch disease
   - Drug reaction (ulcerative, erythema multiforme, lichenoid reaction, TEN)
   - Fungal infection other than candidiasis

- *Cryptococcus neoformans*
- *Histoplasma capsulatum*
- Mucormycosis
- *Aspergillus flavus*
- Neurological
    - Facial palsy
    - Trigeminal neuralgia
- Recurrent aphthous stomatitis
    - Viral infection
    - Cytomegalovirus
    - Molluscum contagiosum
- Clinical feature ranges from asymptomatic infection to severe clinical illness and AIDS
- Patient is generally asymptomatic until CD4 count falls below 500 cells/mm^3 at which patient enter symptomatic HIV infection.
- AIDS is diagnosed when CD4 cells count falls below 200 cells/mm^3.
- Advanced HIV infection—CD4 cell count <50 cells/mm^3 overwhelming opportunistic infection and death.

Q6. Lab diagnosis of HIV:

Ans.
- Specific—ELISA, Western blot, immunoflorescence
    - Antigen detection
    - Polymerase chain reaction test
- Indirect—CD4 and CD8 cell count
    - Lymphopenia
    - Lymph node biopsy
        1. Vital p24 Ag by ELISA—detectable mostly after infection but disappears 8–10 weeks after exposure.
        2. IgG Ab to p24 antigen
        3. Isolation of virus in culture and detection by PCR
        4. CD4 + T cell count: Decrease in peripheral blood while CD8 cell count remains unchanged.

Diseases of Blood and its Oral Manifestations

Q1. What are the normal values of blood components?

Ans. Normal RBC count: 4.5–5.5 million/L

Normal hemoglobin levels:

– Men: 13–18 g/dl

– Women: 11.5–16.5 g/dl

Normal WBC count: 4,000 to 11,000/cu.mm

Normal platelet count: 1.5 to 4.5 lakhs /cu. mm

Red blood cell disorders are

Polycythemia: Abnormal increase in RBC count. Presents as ruddy cyanosis. Purplish discoloration of oral mucosa and lingual varicosities.

Anemia: Abnormal decrease in hemoglobin concentration.

Q2. Classification of anemia.

Ans. A. *Pathophysiologic classification*

    I. Anemia due to increased blood loss

   II. Anemia due to impaired red cell production

     • Iron deficiency anaemia, thalassemia

     • Vitamin B_{12} and/or folic acid deficiency: Megaloblastic anaemia

     • Defect in stem cell proliferation: Aplastic anemia

   III. Anemias due to red cell destruction (hemolytic anemias)

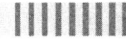

B. *Morphologic classification*
  I. Microcytic, hypochromic, e.g. Iron deficiency anemia , thalassemia and sickle cell anemia
  II. Normocytic, normochromic, e.g. aplastic anemia
  III. Macrocytic, normochromic, e.g. megaloblastic anemia.

Q3. Symptoms of anemia.

Ans. • Pale skin—Pallor

• Easy fatigue and loss of energy

• Unusually rapid heart beat, particularly with exercise

• Shortness of breath and headache, particularly with exercise

• Difficulty concentrating

• Dizziness

• Leg cramps

• Upward curvature of the nails, referred to as *koilonychia*.

Q4. Oral manifestations of anemia.

Ans. • Angular cheilitis

• Glossodynia and atrophic glossitis of tongue: Bald tongue

• Pale oral mucosa

• Oral candidiasis

• Recurrent aphthous stomatitis

• Erythematous mucositis

Q5. Which syndrome is associated with iron deficiency anemia?

Ans. • Plummer-Vinson syndrome. It is also known as Paterson-Kelly syndrome or sideropenic dysphagia.

• It is a rare syndrome with classic triad of dysphagia, iron deficiency anemia and upper esophageal webs or strictures.

- Usually affects middle-aged white women in 4th to 7th decade of life.
- Radiographic examination (barium swallow) of the pharynx shows the presence of webs.
- It is a **premalignant condition**.

Q6. Dental considerations of anemia.

Ans. For patients with extremely low hemoglobin levels, physician consultation prior to surgical treatment is recommended.

When hemoglobin is less than 8 g/dl general anesthesia should be avoided and the potential for clinical bleeding and faulty wound healing should be recognized.

Q7. Causes of hemolytic anemia.

Ans. Hemolytic anemia presents as pallor as well as icterus

- Radiographically presents as **hair-on-end appearance:** Erythroid elements of bone marrow are hyperplastic in attempt to compensate for anemia. Because of enlargement of medullary spaces, trabeculae become more prominent, creating increase in bone radiolucency with prominent lamellar striations.

Etiology

Severe infections and toxins

- Hypersplenism
- Rh factor incompatibility (erythroblastosis foetalis)
- Chronic liver disease
- Tranfusion reactions
- Autoimmune hemolytic disease

Abnormal shape of erythrocytes—hereditary spherocytosis/elliptocytosis

- Erythrocyte enzyme deficiencies (G6PD, pyruvate kinase)

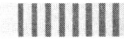

Q8. What are hemoglobinopathies?

Ans. • Sickle cell anemia
   • Thalassemia

Q9. Features of sickle cell anemia.

Ans. Normocytic normochromic anemia with abnormal hemoglobin called HbS in RBCs which are sickle shaped.

• Sickle cell trait—asymptomatic carrier: HbA – α2 β2
• Substitution of valine for glutamic acid at position 6 of beta-globin gene (HbS) α2 β2 valine 6
• During hypoxia sickling of RBCs occurs (*Tactoids*) which leads to stasis of blood vessels and vaso occlusive crisis and increased susceptibility to osteomyelitis.
• Presents as pallor and icterus.
• Radiographically presents as **Step ladder pattern** and hair on end appearance.

Q10. Features of thalassemia.

Ans. • Microcytic hypochromic. Also called Mediterranean anemia
• Group of genetic disorders of hemoglobin synthesis. Characterized by disturbance of alpha (thalessemia major or Cooley's anemia) or beta (thalessemia minor) Hb chain production.

Features

Anemia—Ashen gray pallor, fatigue and weakness and icterus

Expansion of bone marrow. Migration and spacing of upper anterior teeth

Chip—Munk facies or rodent facies and hair on end appearance.

Q11. What is megaloblastic anemia?

Ans. Macrocytic normochromic anemia
Etiology: Vitamin B_{12} deficiency/folic acid deficiency
Intrinsic factor deficiency (Addisonian pernicious anemia)

Features
- Lemon tinted pallor.
- Nerve related disorders
- Angular cheilitis
- Skin pigmentation
- Beefy Red tongue and glossitis/glossodynia / glossopyrosis

Diagnosis by Schilling test

WHITE BLOOD CELL DISORDERS

- Neutrophils provide first line of defence against bacterial invasion and are most abundant.
- Neutrophil counts are raised in bacterial infections.
  - Eosinophils function in antigen antibody reactions and are increased in parasitic infections.
  - Basophils act as mast cells in allergic reactions.
  - Lymphocytes are basically involved in immunity.
  - Granulocytosis : Increase in number of WBCs can result from infection, tissue necrosis, allergic reactions and neoplastic disorders.
  - An elevation up to 30000/ mm^3 with a pronounced left shift and presence of myelocytes, meta-myelocytes and band forms is called a "leukemoid reaction."
  - Granulocytopenia are called neutropenia and the number of neutrophils is reduced to 3000 to 6000/ mm^3 in the peripheral blood Agranulocytosis.
  - Cyclic neutropenia recurs in a regular periodicity of 21 days, persists for 3 to 5 days, and is characterized by infectious events.
  - Agranulocytosis is decrease in WBC count and occurs due to suppression of the bone marrow.

Q12. Features of agranulocytosis:

Ans. • Complication: Infections especially bacterial (Klebsiella, Pseudomonas, Proteus) with decreased signs of inflammation. Swelling and pus are minimal.

- Malaise—headache, discomfort, muscle aches
- Mucosal ulcers — localised clinical signs of infection are decreased due to decreased inflammatory reaction and presence of necrotic slough. Gingivitis and severe periodontitis.
- Fever
- Tachycardia
- Acute pharyngitis, UTI, RTI
- Lymphadenopathy.

Q13. What is Chédiak-Higashi syndrome?

Ans. • Qualitative disorders of WBCs: Decreased chemotactic (lazy leukocyte) and bactericidal activity
- Intact phagocytosis
- Rare autosomal recessive defect with oculocutaneous albinism, neuropathy and severe neutropenia.

Q14. Features of leukemia.

Ans. • Leukemia is a malignant tumor of hematopoietic stem cells characterized by the progressive over production of white blood cells which usually appear in the circulating blood in an immature form at the expense of normal cell production in bone marrow leading to suppression of normal cells causing anemia, thrombocytopenia and a deficiency of normally functioning leukocytes. .
- Type A: Acute and chronic and type B: Lymphocytic and myelogenous.

Etiology
- Radiation and chemicals
- Viruses: Epstein-Barr virus, human T-cell leukemia virus
- Chromosomal abnormality: Philadelphia chromosome
- Genetic disorders

Q15. Oral manifestations of leukemia.

Ans. Pallor, depapillation of tongue and angular cheilitis
Petechiae, ecchymosis, gingival hemorrhage
Gingival enlargement, ANUG, candidiasis, histoplasmosis,
herpes simplex and herpes zoster and non-specific
ulcerations.
- Radiographically, ill-defined patchy radiolucency and
  there may be lamina dura loss and cortical outlines of
  follicles may be effaced.

BLEEDING AND CLOTTING DISORDERS

**Q16. Mention the blood investigations for bleeding
disorder patients:**

Ans. Bleeding time: 1 to 5 mins
Clotting time: 3 to 6 mins
Prothrombin time: 15 to 20 secs
Partial thromboplastin time: 25 to 40 secs
Thrombin time: 9 to 13 secs
INR test : 1 to 1.5

Q17. What is INR?

Ans. International normalized ratio. The INR is a test of blood
clotting, which is primarily used to monitor warfarin
therapy, where the aim is to maintain an elevated INR in
a certain range, e.g. 2.0 to 3.0. The ratio of the sample's
prothrombin time (PT—a measure of clotting), to the
prothrombin time of a normal sample of blood. A result
of 1.0, up to 1.5, is therefore normal.

Q18. Features of hemophilia.

Ans. • Also called by the names "the disease of kings".
Inherited hemorrhagic disorder caused by deficiency
of factor VIII (hemophilia A) or factor IX (hemophilia
B). Hemophilia C is factor XI deficiency. Factor V
deficiency is called parahemophilia.

- X-linked recessive inheritance hence affect males more
  commonly. Female who carry a single mutated gene,
  are generally asymptomatic.

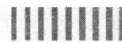

- Deep bleeding into joints and muscles is the hallmark.
- Begins when the child reaches the toddler age.
- Gingival bleeding and petechiae.

Investigations

- Complete hemogram
  a. Hb count—decreased
  b. TLC—normal
  c. DLC—normal
  d. Platelet count—normal
- X- ray of joint
- Factor VIII assay
- Coagulation time—prolonged
- Prothrombin time—usually normal
- Activated partial thromboplastin time—prolonged to 2–3 times

Treatment

- Factor VIII therapy.

10

Systemic Disease and its Dental Considerations

A. CARDIOVASCULAR DISEASE AND HYPERTENSION

Q1. What is hypertension? What is its normal range?

Ans. Hypertension is a condition in which arterial blood pressure is chronically elevated resulting from increased peripheral arteriolar resistance.

Category	Systolic (mm Hg)	Diastolic (mm Hg)
Normal	<120	<80
Prehypertensive	120–139	80–89
Hypertension		
• Stage I	140–159	90–99
• Stage II	>=160	>=100

Q2. What are the symptoms of hypertension?

Ans. • General
  • Headache
  • Dizziness
  • Palpitation
  • Easy fatiguability
  • Symptoms referable to systemic vascular involvement
  • Epistaxis
  • Blurring of vision

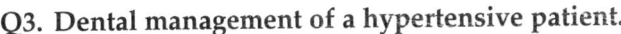

Q3. Dental management of a hypertensive patient.

Ans. • Careful treatment planning, premedication, selection of anaesthesia and determining the duration and the extent of operative procedures.

• Detailed family history of cardiovascular disease, history of hypertension, medications, duration and antihypertensive treatment. Status of thyroid levels, pregnancy and diabetes mellitus.

• Always check BP of every patient especially before extraction and surgical procedures.

• Short, minimally stressful appointments.

• An aspiration should be done before giving anaesthesia.

• It is essential to avoid anxiety and pain, so adequate analgesia must be provided.

• High epinephrine in gingival retraction cords are contraindicated.

• Recommended dose of epinephrine in LA is 0.04 mg which is equal to 4 cartridges of 1:100,000 or 2 cartridges of 1:200,000 in cardiac risk patient.

• Premedication with antianxiety drugs and inhalation of nitrous oxide in anxious patients, e.g. 5 mg diazepam

• Increased risk of bleeding in hypertensive patient.

• Patient position on dental chair is semirecline, if position is flat patient may feel breathless.

• Elective procedures especially those requiring general anaesthesia should be avoided for at least four weeks after MI.

• Avoid corticosteroids as they are known to raise the blood pressure.

Q4. Dental management of bleeding after extraction in a hypertensive patient.

Ans. • Hypertensive patient may have higher bleeding tendency.

• The patient should be calmed down.

- Hemostatic collagen used for wound protection and for control of bleeding.
- Gelatin (e.g. Gelfoam) can be used for control of minor bleeding.
- Bone wax is commonly used for mandibular 3rd molar extractions.
- Cellulose
- Sutures after extractions

Q5. Oral manifestation caused by effects of antihypertensive drugs.

Ans. 1. **Xerostomia:** ACE inhibtors, thiazide diuretics, loop diuretics associated with xerostomia which can cause decay, difficulty in chewing, swallowing, speaking, candidiasis and burning mouth syndrome.

2. **Gingival hyperplasia:** It can be caused by calcium channel blocker, e.g. nifedipine.

3. **Lichenoid reaction:** Many antihypertensives (thiazide diuretics, methyl dopa, etc.) are associated both oral lichenoid reactions.

4. **Loss of taste/taste alterations:** Associated mainly with ACE inhibtors.

5. **Paraesthesia:** Due to drug labetalol

6. **Burning sensation:** Caused by drug captopril.

Q6. Clinical features of ischaemic heart disease.

Ans. • Chest tightness
- Jaw discomfort
- Left arm pain
- Dyspnoea
- Epigastric distress
- Physical exertion (main) particularly in cold weather
- Emotion (anger or anxiety) and stress caused by fear or pain and typically releived by rest.

Q7. **Dental considerations in ischemic heart disease.**

Ans.
- Stress, anxiety, exertion or Pain can provoke angina.
- Short, minimally stressful dental appointments.
- Late morning appointments.
- Excessive dose of LA containing adrenaline to be avoided in patients taking beta-blockers.
- Preoperative glyceryl trinitrate and oral sedation advised sometimes.
- Monitor pulse and BP.
- LA containing adrenaline is contraindicated in IHD (may ppt dysrhythmia)
- Post-angioplasty elective dental care deferred for 6 months, emergency dental care in a hospital setting.
- Patients with by-pass grafts—antibiotic cover against infective endocarditis.
- Patients with vascular stents—no antibiotic cover except during 1st 6 weeks postoperative for emergency dental care.
- More common–severe dental caries and periodontal disease in patients of IHD.

B. RESPIRATORY DISORDERS

Q8. **Clinical features of acute maxillary sinusitis:**

Ans.
- Facial pain on involved side
- Tenderness of teeth
- Headache
- Pain in occipital region if sphenoid sinus and post-ethmoid sinuses are involved
- Purulent nasal discharge
- Fever
- Malaise
- Postnasal drip with fetid breath
- Anosmia

Diagnostic aids
- PNS view
- CT
- MRI

Q9. Management of acute maxillary sinusitis.

Ans.
- Antibiotics (amoxicillin, cephalosporins)
- Topical or oral decongestants
- Steam inhalation

Q10. Oral manifestations of viral upper respiratory tract infections.

Ans.
- Small round erythematous macular lesions on soft palate
- Decreased salivary flow due to side effects of decongestants.

Q11. Oral findings pharyngitis and tonsillitis:

Ans.
- EBV leads to infectious mononucleosis—tonsillo-pharyngitis
- Lymphadenopathy
- Fever, fatigue
- Hepatosplenomegaly
- Elevated liver enzymes
- Coxsackievirus causing herpangina causes ulcers 2–3 mm on anterior tonsillar pillars, uvula, soft palate
- Coxsackievirus causing Hand-foot and -mouth disease causing ulcers on tongue and oral mucosa and vesicles on palms and soles. Small yellow white nodules on anterior tonsillar pillars characterize lymphonodular pharyngitis.
- Measles producing Koplik's spots on inner aspect of lower lip and buccal mucosa
- Streptococcal pharyngitis causing tonsillitis, fever, beefy red uvula and oral petechiae

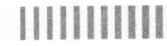

Q12. Oral health considerations in respiratory tract diseases.

Ans. • Oral dryness—due to decongestants.
- Increased susceptibility to gingivitis in mouth breathers

Q13. Oral health considerations in COPD.

Ans. • Blue bloaters (cyanosis)
- Pink puffers
- Since these patients may be under treatment with Heparin they may have haemostatic complications. Dental care can safely be provided for patients. With prothrombin times of up to 20 seconds.

Q14. Clinical features of bronchial asthma.

Ans. • Hallmark—recurrent reversible airflow limitation and airway hyperresponsiveness
- Wheezing
- Coughing
- Dyspnea
- Chest tightness
  Chest tightness which worsens at night.
  Diagnostic aids
- Allergen skin testing
- Chest radiography

Q15. Oral health considerations in bronchial asthma.

Ans. • Numerous dental products and materials have been associated with exacerbation of asthma
- Nasal respiratory obstruction resulting in *mouth breathing leads* to development of long and tapered facial form, increased lower facial height and narrow maxillary arch
- Oral manifestations include candidiasis, decreased salivary flow, *increased calculus, gingivitis,* periodontal disease and caries incidence.

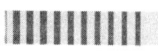

Q16. Considerations and recommendations for administering dental care to asthmatic patients.

Ans. • Fluoride supplements
- Rinse mouth after use of inhalers
- Reinforcement of oral hygiene
- Antifungal medications
- Steroid prophylaxis
- Stress reducing techniques
- Appointments for late morning or later in day
- Have oxygen and bronchodilators
- Use of rubber dams
- Care while using suction tips
- During an acute asthmatic attack, i.e. status asthamaticus, dental procedure should be discontinued and if no improvement noticed administer epinephrine subcutaneously.

C. DIABETES MELLITUS

Q17. Classify diabetes mellitus (DM).

Ans. • Type 1 DM ("insulin dependent DM")
- Type 2 DM ("non insulin dependent DM ")
- DM occurring secondary to genetic disorders, diseases or injury to the pancreas and other endocrine diseases
- Gestational diseases.

Q18. Physiology of blood glucose.

Ans. • In healthy persons, plasma glucose levels are 63–144 mg/dl.
- Principal organ of glucose homeostasis is the liver, which absorb and store glucose in post-absorptive state between meals and meet the energy needs.
- Liver is also site of gluconeogenesis, whereby glucose molecule is derived from fat, muscle glycogen and protein.

Q19. Functions of insulin:

Ans.
- Insulin is the key hormone involved in storage and controlled release of energy.
- It is produced by beta cells of pancreas.
- In the fasting state, insulin functions to regulate the release of glucose by liver and in the postprandial state it facilitates the uptake of glucose by fat and muscle.

Q20. Counter regulatory hormone of insulin which increases blood glucose level?

Ans. Counter-regulatory hormones—glucagon, catecholamines, GH, thyroid hormone and glucocorticoids.

Q21. Pathophysiology of DM.

Ans.

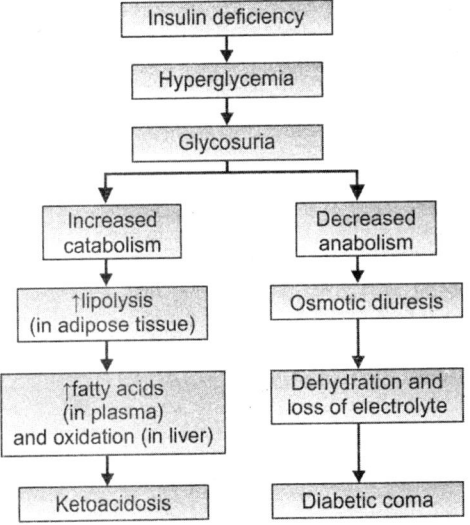

Q22. Pathogenesis of type 1 and type 2 diabetes mellitus.

Ans. Type 1 diabetes mellitus:
- Increase blood glucose level.
- Glucose as main energy source but cannot get absorbed.
- Polyuria and polydipsia.

Type 2 diabetes mellitus:
- Decrease in number of insulin receptor.

Q23. Complications of type 1 and 2 diabetes mellitus.

Ans. • Type 1 diabetes mellitus: Diabetic ketoacidosis
- Type 2 diabetes mellitus: Electrolyte imbalance and acidosis.

Q24. Signs and symptoms of undiagnosed diabetes mellitus (DM).

Ans. • Polydipsia
- Polyuria
- Polyphagia
- Unexplained weight loss
- Weakness, malaise
- Nocturnal enuresis
- Irritability
- Dry mouth
- Chronic skin infection
- Ketoacidosis
- Changes in vision
- Pruritis
- Impotence
- Postural hypertension
- Initially asymptomatic

Q25. Normal fasting and non-fasting blood glucose level.

Ans.

Criterion	Normal	Impaired fasting glucose	Diabetes mellitus
Fasting glucose	< 110 mg/dl	110–126 mg/dl	≥126 mg/dl
2 hours post-prandial glucose	>140 mg/dl	140–200 mg/dl	≥200 mg/dl

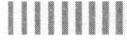

Q26. Vascular complications associated with diabetes mellitus (DM).

Ans. Disorders such as hypertension and dyslipidemia, commonly seen in people with DM increase the risk of microvascular and macrovascular complications. The vascular complication result from atherosclerosis and microangiopathy increased lipid deposition and atheroma formation are seen in larger blood vessels along with increased thickness of arterial walls proliferation of endothelial cells,alteration in endothelial basement membrane and changes in the function of endothelial cells induce microvascular damage.

Q27. Oral manifestation and complications of diabetes mellitus.

Ans. 1. Candidiasis
2. Periodontal disease, multiple periodontal abscesses.
3. Odontogenic related soft tissue infection and cellulitis
4. Due hyposalivation increased risk of dental caries, particularly smooth surface caries, oral dryness, atrophy of oral mucosa and increased frequency and severity in all clinical forms of candida infection.
5. Xerostomia
6. Burning mouth syndrome and bilateral sialosis
7. Angular cheilitis
8. Lichenoid drug reaction.

Q28. Precautions before undertaking dental surgical procedure in a diabetic patient.

Ans. • Check the patient's blood glucose level.
• Hypoglycemic patient can be provided with replacement sugar.
• For a conscious patient this can be into form of glucose drink (150 ml carbonated lemonade, 2 teaspoons of table sugar or preferably glucose in water) followed by a rechecking their blood glucose level .
• If patient exhibits deteriorating level of consciousness, then IM administration of glucagon.

Q29. Classic signs of DM.

Ans. • Polyuria
  • Polydipsia
  • Polyphagia
  • Weight loss
  • Either disturbed vision or peripheral neuropathy.
  • Advanced periodontal disease and multiple perio-
    dontal abscesses.

Q30. Antidiabetic drugs.

Ans. • Sulfonylurea
  • Biguanides
  • Alfa-glucoside
  • Insulin therapy

Q31. Dental management of diabetes mellitus patient.

Ans. Scheduling of visits
  • Morning appointment
  • Do not coincide with peak activity
  Diet
  • Ensure that the patient has eaten normally and taken
    medications as usual
  Blood glucose monitoring
  • Measured before beginning (<70 mg/dl)
  Prophylactic antibiotics
  • Established infection
  • Preoperation contamination wound
  • Major surgery of diabetic patient in dental office
    – Epinephrine is not contraindicated in dental
      treatment of diabetic patients
    – Because it helps promotes better dental anasthesia
      and adequate pain control and stress reduction
    – Common emergency is hypoglycemia, which may
      result in seizures and loss of consciousness .
    – To avoid hypoglycemic attacks:

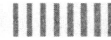

- Oral carbohydrate
- Subcutaneous glucagon
  - To avoid hyperglycemia
- Pretreatment anxiety should be reduced by sedation
- Pain during procedures can be avoided by potent anesthesia
  - Check for blood glucose with glucometer.
  - The *"golden rule"* is that manage the patients as if they are hypoglycemic until proven otherwise.

Q32. Factors that increase risk of hypoglycemia.

Ans.
- Skipping or delaying of food intake
- Injection of too much insulin
- Injection of insulin into tissue with high blood flow
- Alcohol consumption
- Anxiety, stress
- Inability to recognize symptoms of hypoglycemia
- Denial of warning signs and symptoms

Q33. Difference between hyperglycemia and hypoglycemia.

Ans.

Hyperglycemia	Hypoglycemia
• It refers to an excess of glucose in blood stream	• It refers to a deficiency of glucose in blood stream
• Blood sugar level rises more than 130 mg/dl	• Blood sugar level drops less than 70 mg/dl
• Can be caused by non-compliance of anti-glycemic agents	• Can be caused by excessive intake of anti-glycemic agents beyond the prescribed dose
• Commonest complication is hyperosmolar, hyperglycemic, non-ketotic syndrome	• Commonest complication is diabetic ketoacidosis
• Dry and dehydrated skin	• Sweating present. Skin is pale, cold and clammy
• Weak pulse	• Rapid and strong pulse
• Fruity acetone breath	• Absent
• Hyperventilation present	• Normal

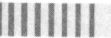

D. GIT AND LIVER DISEASE

GIT Disease Includes

- Inflammatory bowel diseases
  Ulcerative colitis there is rectal bleeding with diarrhoea and crampy pain.
  Crohn's disease—inflammation of small and large intestine involving all layers of gut. Anemia, abdominal pain, nausea, vomiting, weight loss.
- Peptic ulcer disease
- Gastro-oesophageal reflux disorder (GERD)
- Malabsorption
- Eating disorders, e.g. anorexia bulimia nervosa

Q34. Oral manifestation of ulcerative colitis.

Ans. • There are features of anemia.
  - **Major and minor aphthous ulcers**
  - Pyostomatitis vegetans: A purulent inflammation of mouth may occur
  - Ulcerative colitis patients also can develop hairy leukoplakia, a lesion more commonly associated with human immunodeficiency virus (HIV) disease.

Q35. Oral manifestations of Crohn's disease:

Ans. • Diffuse swelling of the lips and face
  - Persistent ulcers
  - Cobblestone mucosal architecture
  - Indurated polypoid tag-like lesions in the vestibule.

Q36. Dental management of inflammatory bowel diseases.

Ans. 1. Frequent preventive and routine dental care to monitor oral health .
  2. Evaluation of hypothalamus-pituitary adrenocortical function
  3. Diagnosis of oral inflammatory or granulomatous lesions
  4. Palliative rinses and topical steroid therapy symptomatic oral lesions.

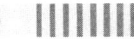

Q37. Oral manifestations of peptic ulcer.

Ans. • Xerostomia
- Altered taste perception
- Mucosal pallor
- Thrombocytopenia and gingival bleeding
- Agranulocytosis causing mucosal ulcerations and necrotising stomatitis
- Susceptibility to fungal disease and bacterial disease.

Q38. Dental management of peptic ulcer disease:

Ans. • Minimize stress
- Selective usage of analgesics
- Check for count before any surgical procedure
- Frequent recall and oral prophylaxis is recommended
- Avoidance of tetracycline in patients taking aluminium antacids.

Q39. Oral manifestation of gastroesophageal reflux disease (GERD).

Ans. 1. Dysgeusia (altered taste)

2. Esophageal stricture and fibrosis

3. Mucosal atrophy

4. Xerostomia

5. Erosion

6. Mucosal erythema

Q40. Dental management of gastroesophageal reflux disease (GERD):

Ans. • $NaHCO_3$ mouth rinses to minimize dysguesia due to acid reflux .
- Topical flouride application to ensure optimal mineralisation
- Salivary substitute may be prescribed
- Patients should be advised to have adequate amount of fluid intake

Q41. Oral manifestations of malabsorption:

Ans. • Inflamed "beefy red" tongue
- Glossitis and glossodynia
- Angular cheilitis
- Recurrent aphthous ulcer

Q42. Oral manifestations of eating disorders/bulimia.

Ans. • Erosion of lingual surfaces of maxillary anterior teeth
- Increased risk of caries
- Parotid gland enlargement
- Dentinal hypersensitivity—teeth sensitive to thermal changes.

Q43. Oral manifestations of liver diseases:

Ans. • Oral candidiasis
- Angular cheilitis
- Atrophic glossitis
- Petechiae
- Lichen planus
- Oral metastases of hepatocellular carinoma primarily manifest as hemorrhagic expanding masses located in the premolar and ramus region of the mandible.

Q44. Dental management of a patient with liver disease:

Ans. 1. **Protection for the practitioner:** Difficult or impossible to identify carriers of HBV, HCV. Most carriers are unaware that they have had hepatitis.
   – HBV vaccination
   – Standard precautions
   – Post-exposure prophylaxis

2. **Metabolism of dental drugs:**
   Local anesthetics: Lidocaine, prilocaine, articaine
   Analgesics: Aspirin, acetaminophen, narcotics, morphine
   Sedative: Benzodiazepines
   Antibiotics: Ampicillin, tetracycline, metronidazole, vancomycin.

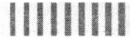

3. **Impaired hemostasis:**

Clotting factors II, VII, IX and X are impaired because of liver disease, hence such patients can present with petechiae and echymosis. There can be prolonged bleeding after extraction.

E. RENAL DISORDERS

Q45. Functions of the kidneys:

Ans. • Excretion of metabolic waste

• Blood pressure control

• Acid–base balance and electrolyte regulation

• Vitamin D activation

• Renin secretion and the regulation of volume and composition of extracellular fluid.

• Erythropoietin production—it is produced and released by the kidneys in response to decreased oxygen tension in the renal blood supply that is created by the loss of red blood cells. Its deficiency leads to anemia in renal failure.

Q46. Systemic disturbances in renal disease.

Ans. 1. GIT: Nausea, vomiting, anorexia, ammonical taste and smell, stomatitis, parotitis

2. Neuromuscular: Headache, peripheral neuropathy, paralysis, seizures

3. Haematological: Due to anemia there is a decreased erythropoietin production, and lymphocytopenia.

   Increased bleeding tendency and haemostatic problems are usually observed in chronic renal failure patients due to abnormal platelet adhesion and aggregation, decrease of platelet factor III and alteration in prothrombin metabolism.

4. Endocrine: Secondary hyperthyroidism, impaired growth and development

5. Cardiovascular: Arterial hypertension, congestive heart failure, pericarditis, arrhythmias.

6. Effects on bone: Bone resorption and osteitis fibrosa due to decreased serum calcium and calcitriol levels. Delayed growth or rickets (renal osteodystrophy).

7. Delayed tooth eruption.

Q47. Oral manifestations of renal disease:

Ans. • Pallor

• Ammonical breath

• Uremic stomatitis: An acute rise in blood urea nitrogen (BUN) may result in uremic stomatitis which may appear as erythemapultaceous form (soft, when pressed indentation is left) characterized by red mucosa covered with a thick exudate and a pseudomembrane.

• Xerostomia

• Periodontal disease

• Delayed healing

• Bleeding from gums and hemostatic defects (petechiae and ecchymosis)

• Tooth erosion (secondary to regurgitation associated with dialysis)

• Gingival overgrowth in kidney transplant patient due to cyclosporine

• Oral hairy leukoplakia in kidney transplant patients.

Q48. Radiographic features of renal disease:

Ans. • Demineralization of bone

• Loss of bony trabeculation

• Ground-glass appearance

• Loss of lamina dura

• Giant cell lesions, "brown tumors"

• Socket sclerosis

• Pulpal narrowing and calcification

• Tooth mobility

• Bone osteodystrophy

Q49. Dental considerations in renal disease:

Ans. 1. Determine dialysis schedule and treat one day after dialysis.
2. Consult with patient's nephrologist for recent laboratory tests and discussion of antibiotic prophylaxis.
3. Evaluate patient for hypertension/hypotension.
4. Institute preoperative hemostatic aids when appropriate. Use adjunctive hemostatic aids during oral/periodontal surgical procedures.
5. Determine underlying cause of renal failure (underlying disease may affect provision of care).
6. Obtain routine annual dental radiographs to establish presence and follow manifestations of renal osteodystrophy.
7. Consider routine serology for HBV, HCV, and HIV antibody.
8. Eliminate potential sources of infection/bacteremia.
9. Maintain patient in a comfortable uncramped position in the dental chair.
10. Allow patient to walk or stand intermittently during long procedures
11. Encourage meticulous home care.
12. Consider use of postoperative antibiotics for traumatic procedures.
13. Avoid use of respiratory-depressant drugs in presence of severe anemia.
14. Adjust dosages of postoperative medications according to extent of renal failure.
15. Consider sedative premedication for patients with hypertension
16. Drugs excreted by the kidney should be given with caution in renal diseases. The list is as follows
    Antibiotics: Penicillins, cephalosporins, aminoglycosides, tetracycline
    Beta blockers, diuretics digoxin, procainamide, cimetidine, ranitidine.

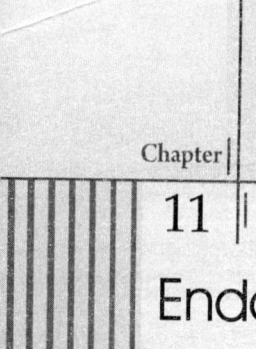

11

Endocrine Disorders and their Oral Considerations

Q1. What is hyperthyroidism? What are its clinical features?

Ans. Decreased level of TSH .
Increased level of T3, T4

Causes
- Thyroid nodules
- Thyroiditis
- Graves' disease
- Medication

Clinical symptoms
- Exopthalmos
- Tremors
- Weight loss
- Heat intolerance—moist clammy skin
- Hair loss
- Anxiety
- Goiter

Q2. Oral and dental manifestations of hyperthyroidism:

Ans.
- Accelerated Dental eruptions
- Burning mouth syndrome
- Increased caries
- Periodontal disease
- Maxillary and mandibular osteoporosis

Q3. Dental considerations of hyperthyroidism.

Ans. • Brief, stress free appointments.

• No LA and retraction cord with epinephrine for uncontrolled HTN

• Sialolith

• Susceptibility to infection

• Avoid iodised salt

Q4. What is hypothyroidism? What are its clinical features?

Ans. • Decreased T3, T4

• Increased TSH

Causes and types

• Cretinism—deficency or absence of thyroid hormone in childhood resulting in dwarfism and mental retardation.

• Myxedema, e.g. autoimmune Hashimoto's thyroiditis

Clinical symptoms

• Fatigue, lethargy

• Weight gain

• Puffiness of face and eyelids

• Cold intolerance (dry cool skin)

• Thin hair, brittle nails

• Goiter

• Dysmenorrhea

Q5. Oral and dental manifestations of hypothyroidism.

Ans. Oral manifestations

• Delayed eruption

• Salivary gland enlargement

• Macroglossia, glossitis and dysguesia

• Delayed healing

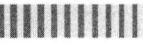

Q6. Dental considerations of hypothyroidism.

Ans. Avoid sedatives like diazepam and narcotic as they cause respiratory and cardiac depression.

Q7. What is hypoparathyroidism? What are its features?

Ans. It is defined as decreased function of parathyroid gland with *under-production* of parathyroid hormone which leads to low level of calcium in the blood (hypocalcemia).

Symptoms
- Tingling of finger tips
- Dryness
- Brittle nails
- Twitching
- Fish mouth and trismus
- Chvostek's sign and Trousseau's sign are positive

Q8. Dental manifestations of hypoparathyroidism:

Ans.
- Enamel hypoplasia
- Pulp calcifications
- Shortened roots
- Hypodontia
- Delayed development of teeth
- Chronic candidiasis.

Q9. Dental considerations of hypoparathyroidism.

Ans. More susceptibility to caries.

Q10. What is hyperparathyroidism? What are its features?

Ans.
- An excess of serum PTH increases bone remodeling but tips the balance between osteoblastic and osteoclastic activity in favor of osteoclastic resorption.
- PTH increases the renal tubular reabsorption of calcium and renal production of the active vitamin D metabolite 1,25 (OH) 2D.
- The net result is increase in serum calcium levels, i.e hypercalcemia.

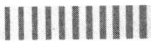

Types

Primary: Results from an adenoma of one of the four parathyroid glands, resulting in excess of PTH production

Secondry: Results from a compensatory increase in the output of PTH response to hypocalcemia, e.g. in kidney failure and vitamin D deficiency

Symptoms

- Fragile *bone* (easily fractures)
- Kidney *stone*
- Get tired easily (*moan*)
- Abdominal pain (*groan*)
- Depression

Q11. Dental manifestations of hyperparathyroidism.

Ans.
- Widened pulp chambers
- Alteration in eruptions
- Malocclusion
- Generalised loss of lamina dura

Q12. Radiographic features of hyperparathyroidism:

Ans.
- Brown's tumor.
- **Generalised loss of lamina dura.**
- Pepper pot skull and ground glass appearance
- Salt and pepper appearance.
- Erosions of bone from the subperiosteal surfaces of the phalanges of the hand.
- Osteitis fibrosa cystica is seen in advanced cases as localized regions of bone loss.
- Radiopaque teeth standing out in radiolucent jaws.

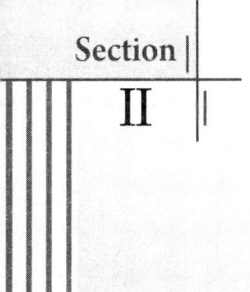

Section II

Radiology

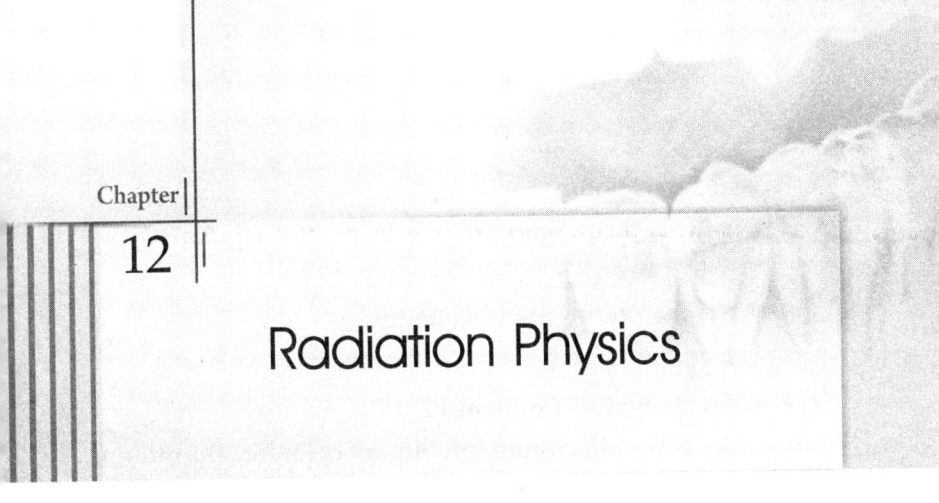

Chapter 12

Radiation Physics

Who Discovered X-rays?

Sir Wilhelm Conrad Roentgen first discovered X-rays on November 1895. He was working with cathode ray tube in laboratory, when first time he observed a fluorescent glow of crystals on a table near his tube.

Q1. Define radiation.

Ans. Radiation is the transmission of energy through space and matter.

Q2. What are the two types of nature of radiation?

Ans. Particulate and electromagnetic.

Q3. What are beta particles of particulate radiation?

Ans. Beta particles are electrons emitted by radioactive nuclei.

Q4. Write the alpha particles of particulate radiation?

Ans. Alpha particles are helium nuclei consisting of two proton and two neutrons.

Q5. What is linear energy transfer (LET)?

Ans. The rate of loss of energy from a particle as it moves along its track through matter (tissue) is its linear energy transfer.

Q6. Define electromagnetic radiation?

Ans. Electromagnetic radiation is the movement of energy through space as a combination of electric and magnetic fields.

Q7. What are photons?

Ans. Quantum theory consider electromagnetic radiation as small bundles of energy called photons.

Q8. Write the unit of photon energy.

Ans. The unit of photon energy is the electronic volt (eV).

Q9. Write the parts of tube head.

Ans. X-ray tube, oil, collimator, aiming cylinder, aluminum filter and power supply are the part of tube head.

Q10. What are the X-ray tubes?

Ans. All medical and dental X-ray tubes are called Coolidge tubes.

Q11. Why are X-ray tube called Coolidge tubes?

Ans. Because they follow the original design made by WC Coolidge, introduced in 1913.

Q12. Write the components of X-ray tube.

Ans. Electronic focusing cup, cathode (–), tube Window, anode (+), copper stem, glass envelope, tungsten target, filament and electric supply.

Q13. What is tube current?

Ans. The tube current is the flow of electrons through the tube, that is, from the filament to anode and then back to the filament through the wiring of the power supply.

Q14. What is function of tube voltage?

Ans. A high voltage is required between the anode and cathode to generate X-rays. An autotransformer converts the primary voltage from the input source into the secondary voltage.

Q15. What is duty cycle?

Ans. Duty cycle relates to the frequency with which successive exposures can be made. The heat storage capacity for anodes of dental diagnostic tube is approximately 20 k HU.

Heat units (HU) = kVp × mA × seconds

Q16. What are the methods of Production of X-rays?
Or
How are X-rays produced?

Ans. 1. Bremsstrahlung: If a high-speed electron directly hits the nucleus of a target atom, all its kinetic energy is transformed into a single X-ray photon. The closer, the high-speed electron approaches the nuclei, the greater is the electrostatic attraction on the electron, the breaking effect, and the energy of the resulting bremsstrahlung photons.

2. Characteristic Radiation: Characteristic radiation occurs when an electron from the filament displaces as electron from a shell of a tungsten target atom thereby ionizing the atom. Characteristic radiation from the K shell occurs only above 70 kVp with a tungsten target and occurs as discrete increments compared with bremsstrahlung radiation. This type of radiation is only a minor source of radiation from an X-ray tube.

Q17. Factors controlling the X-ray beam:

Ans. Tube Current (mA): The quantity of radiation produced by an X-ray tube is directly proportional to the tube current (mA).

Tube voltage (kVp): Increasing the kVp, increases the potential difference between the cathode and anode, thus the target.

1. The number of photons generated,
2. Their mean energy, and
3. Their maximal energy.

The term **beam quality** refers to the mean energy of an X-ray beam.

Filtration: The inherent filtration of most X-ray machines ranges from the equivalent of 0.5 to 2 mm of aluminum.

Collimation: Dental X-ray beams are usually collimated to a circle 2¾ inches (7 cm) in diameter.

Collimator absorbs about 90% of the X-ray photons and 10% of the photons pass through the patient and reach the film.

Q 18. What is inverse-square law?

Ans. The intensity (I) of an X-ray beam at a given point depends inversely on the distance (D) of the measuring device from the focal spot. Therefore, changing the distance between the X-ray tube and patient has a marked effect on beam intensity.

$$\frac{i_1}{i_2} = \frac{(D_2)^2}{(D_1)^2}$$

Q19. What is line focus principle?

Ans. This principle is used to reduce the effective area of the focal spot. The anode is angulated by 20 degrees which alters the actual focal spot size (3 × 3 mm) to effective focal spot size (3 × 1 mm).

Q20. What is total filtration?

Ans. Total filtration = Inherent filtration + added filtration
Inherent filtration by—oil circulating in the tube
Added filtration—aluminium filter placed in the tube head

Q21. Which are the various methods of dissipation of heat to maintain the temperature of the X-ray tube?

Ans. Cooling of the tube can be achieved by oil, using rotating anode and by angulation of anode.

Q22. Which are the different types of scattering?

Ans. 1. Coherent scattering,
2. Photoelectric absorption, and
3. Compton scattering. In addition, about 9% of the primary photons pass through the patient without interaction.

Coherent scattering: Coherent scattering (also known as classical, elastic, or Thompson scattering) may occur when a low-energy incident photon (less than 10 keV) passes near an outer electron of an atom which has a low binding energy.

This interaction account for only about 8% of the total number of interactions (per exposure) in dental examination.

Photoelectric absorption: An incident photon collides with a bound electron in an atom of the absorbing medium.

About 30% of photons absorbed from a dental X-ray beam are absorbed by the photoelectric process.

The frequency of photoelectric interaction varies directly with the third power of the atomic number of the absorber.

Compton scattering: About 62% of photons that are absorbed from a dental X-ray beam are absorbed by this process.

- The probability of a compton interaction is directly proportional to the electron density of the absorber.
- In a dental X-ray beam approximately 62% of the photons undergo Compton scattering.
- Approximately 30% of the scattered photons formed during a dental X-ray exposure exits through the patient's head.

Q23. What are various units of measurement of X-rays exposure?

Ans. Exposure: The SI unit of exposure is air kerma, an acronym for kinetic energy released in matter. Traditional unit—Roentgen (R)

Absorbed dose: Absorbed dose is a measure of the energy absorbed by any type of ionizing radiation per unit mass of any type of matter. SI unit—Gy, Traditional unit—rad

Equivalent dose: Absorbed dose (H_T) is used to compare the biologic effects of different types of radiation to a tissue or organ. SI unit—Seivert, Traditional unit-rem (roentgen equiralent man)

Effective dose: The effective dose (E) is used to estimate the risk in humans. SI unit—Sv (seivert), Traditional unit—rem

Radioactivity: It measures the decay rate of sample of radioactive material. SI unit—Becquerel. Traditional unit—curie

Chapter
13

Radiation Biology

Q1. What are biologic effects of radiation?

Ans. a. Deterministic effects (dose dependent) are those effects in which the severity of response is proportional to the dose. Deterministic effects have a dose threshold below which the response is not seen (example: Oral changes after radiation therapy).

b. Stochastic effects (dose independent) are those for which the probability of the occurrence of a change, rather than its severity, is dose dependent (example: Radiation induced cancer-greater exposure of a person to radiation increases the probability of cancer but not its severity).

Q2. What the direct and indirect effects of radiation?

Ans. **Direct effect:** Direct alteration of biologic molecules (rH, where r is the molecule and H is a hydrogen atom) by ionizing radiation begins with absorption of energy by the biologic molecule and formation of unstable free radicals. Approximately one-third of the biologic effects of X-ray exposure result from direct effects.

Indirect effect: Indirect effect are those in which hydrogen and hydroxyl free radicals, produced by the action of radiation on water, interact with organic molecules.

Q3. How is water affected by radiation?

Ans. Water is the predominant molecule in biologic systems. A complex series of chemical changes occurs in water after exposure to ionizing radiation. Collectively these reactions result in radiolysis of water.

Q4. **What are the components affected by radiation in a cell?**

Ans. Cell components like nucleus, chromosomes and cytoplasm are affected by radiation.

Q5. **Which are the various cell types as per radio-sensitivity?**

Ans. According to french radiobiologists Bergonie and Tribondeau:

1. *Vegetative intermitotic cells are the most radio-sensitive:* Early precursor cells, such as those in the spermatogenic or erythroblastic series, and basal cells of the oral mucous membrane.

2. *Differentiating intermitotic cells:* These are somewhat less radiosensitive than vegetative intermitotic cells, e.g. inner enamel epithelium of developing teeth, cells of the hematopoietic series.

3. *Multipotential connective tissue cells:* They have intermediate radiosensitivity, e.g. vascular endo-thelial cells, fibroblasts.

4. Reverting postmitotic cells are generally radio-resistant because they divide infrequently. Acinar and ductal cells of the salivery glands and pancreas. Parenchymal cells of the liver, kidney, and thyroid.

5. *Fixed postmitotic cells:* These are most resistant to the direct action of radiation, e.g. neurons striated muscle cells, squamous epithelial cells.

Q6. **Response of cells to radiation depends on which factors?**

Ans. **They are:** Radiation dose, dose rate, presence of oxygen, and linear energy transfer.

Q7. **What are the effects of radiation therapy (therapeutic radiation) on oral cavity?**

Ans. The changes can be:
- **Oral mucous membrane:** After 2 weeks of therapy redness and inflammation of mucosa is seen called mucositis. It usually heals after two months.

- **Taste buds:** Loss of taste sensation during second or third week of radiotherapy.
- **Salivary glands:** Reduced salivary flow or xerostomia beyond 60 Gy.
- **Teeth:** Radiation during development can affect the growth. If it precedes calcification, can destroy tooth bud. Premature eruption or altered root formation may also seen.
- **Radiation caries:** Due to reduced salivary flow, there is lack of cleansing action of saliva and development of caries. This is widespread form of caries affecting all tooth surfaces leading to loss of crown structure.
- **Bone:** Due to hypoxia, hypovascularity and hypocellularity osteoradionecrosis of bone occurs.

Q8. What is acute radiation syndrome?

Ans. It is a collection of signs and symptoms experienced by individuals after whole body exposure to radiation. According to dose, symptoms vary (as per involvement of the system)

Dose (Gy)	Manifestations
1–2	Prodromal symptoms
2–4	Mild haematopoetic symptoms
4–7	Severe hematopoetic symptoms
7–15	Gastrointestinal symptoms
50	CVS and CNS symptoms

Radiation caries: This is also called radiation-induced caries which is a late complication of radiotherapy. This condition can lead to a complete loss of teeth gradually. Within a year may it leads to total destruction of originally healthy dentition as it usually has a rapid onset and quick progress. Radiation caries located around the necks of the teeth and typically affecting more than one surface is called *caries circularis*. The teeth located in the irradiated areas are discoloured, brownish, exhibit changes in translucency, and become brittle and prone to fracture.

It is classified as:

Type 1 affecting the cervical aspect of the teeth and extending along the cementoenamel junction.

Type 2 presents with demineralized and worn occlusal surfac s.

Type 3 presents as color changes in the dentin. The crown is dark brown/black, along with occlusal wear.

Radiographic presentation: Radiolucent shadows appearing at necks of the teeth usually on the mesial and distal aspects.

Radiation Safety and Protection

Q1. Which are the sources of radiation exposure?

Ans. Natural and artificial. Annual effective dose from these sources is 3.6 mSv.

Q2. What is equivalent dose (Sv)?

Ans. A quantity that expresses all kinds of radiation on a common scale, is defined as the sum of the products of the absorbed dose in grays and the radiation weighting factor.

Q3. Enlist few natural sources of radiation.

Ans. **External:** Cosmic, terrestrial
Internal: Radion, other

Q4. Enlist few artificial sources of radiation.

Ans. **Medical:** X-ray diagnosis, nuclear medicine
Consumer Products: Occupational, nuclear fuel cycle, fallout, miscellaneous.

Q5. Which factors affect the exposure to x-radiation?

Ans. Choice of equipment, choice of technique, operation of equipment, and processing and interpretation of the radiographic image.

Q6. How much should be focal spot to film distance to reduce amount of radiation to the patient?

Ans. a. 20 cm (8 inches) and
b. 41 cm (16 inches).

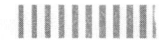

Q7. Position indicating device (PID) helps in reducing X-ray exposure. How?

Ans. PID limits the size of the X-ray beam (even more than required by law) eventually significantly reducing patient exposure.

Q8. What is collimator?

Ans. It is a metallic barrier with an aperture in the middle used to restrict the size and shape of the X-ray beam and the volume of the tissue irradiated. So it helps to improve image quality.

Type of collimators are:
- Rectangular—3.5 × 4.4 cm
- Circular—7 cm

Q9. Rectangular PID is advantageous because:

Ans. Reduces the area of the patient's skin surface to exposure by 60% over that of a round (7 cm) PID.

Q10. Collimators are made of:

Ans. Lead

Q11. Filters are made of:

Ans. Aluminum

Q12. How does filtration help in reduction of radiation exposure?

Ans. When an X-ray beam is filtered with 3 mm of aluminum, the surface exposure is reduced to about 20% of that with no filtration. Low energy photons which have little penetrating power are absorbed by filter without loss of radiologic information.

Minimum half-value layer

Measured X-ray tube voltage (kVp)	Minimum half-value layer (mm Al)
30 to 70	1.5
71	2.1
80	2.3
90	2.5
100	2.7

Q13. What is half-value layer?

Ans. Federal government has designated the specific amount of filtration required for dental X-ray machines operating at various kilovoltages. These quantities, expressed as beam quality (half-value layer: HVL).

Q14. What is position and distance rule?

Ans. The operator should stand at least 6 feet from the patient, at an angle of 90 to 135° to the central ray of the, beam. This rule helps in reduction of X-ray intensity and deviation of scatter radiation to head of the patient.

Q15. Enumerate precautions for operator as a measure for radiation protection.

Ans. 1. Position behind a suitable barrier or wall during exposure of the film.

2. In a radiation area,walls must be of sufficient density or 9-inch thickness that the exposure to non-occupationally exposed individuals is no greater than 100 uGy per week.

3. Follow position-and-distance rule.

4. The operator should never hold films in place. Ideally, film-holding instruments should be used.

5. Neither the operator nor patient should hold the radiographic tube housing during the exposure. Suspension arms should be adequately maintained to prevent housing movement and drift.

6. Personnel-monitoring devices, commonly referred to as film badges should be used.

Q16. What is ALARA?

Ans. It states that the radiation dose should be; as low as reasonably achievable.

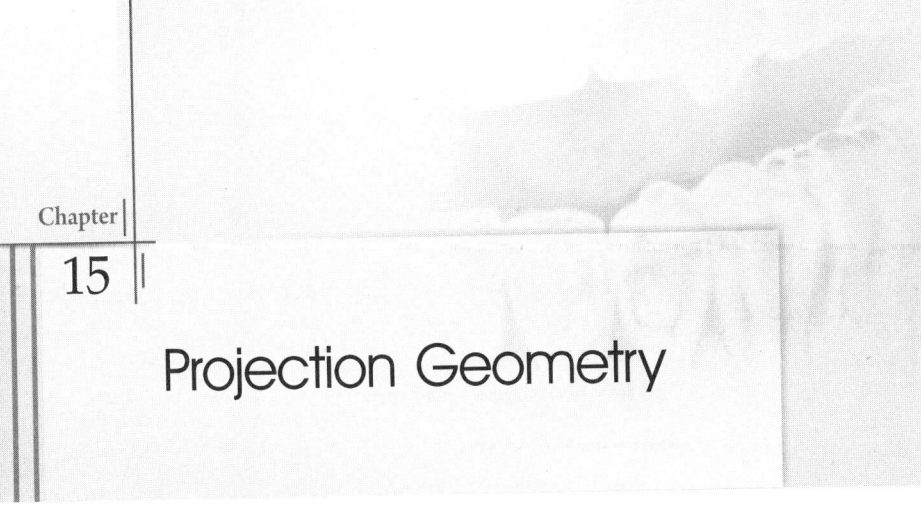

Projection Geometry

Q1. Define ideal radiograph.

Ans. HM Worth—An ideal radiograph has desired density and overall darkness which shows the part completely without distortion with maximum details and with right amount of contrast to make that detail fully apparent.

Q2. What are the characteristics of an ideal radiograph?

Ans. It should have optimum density, contrast, sharpness, resolution and anatomic accuracy of image with adequate coverage of the anatomic region of interest.

Q3. What is umbra?

Ans. It is defined as that part of the shadow when all light is absorbed or area of total darkness.

Q4. What is penumbra?

Ans. It is that part of the shadow of an object which is larger than a point and yet represents a single point of the object. It is thus the unsharpness of the image.

Q5. What are the principles of projection geometry?

Ans. They are:
1. The source of radiation (effective focal spot) should be as small as possible.
2. The distance between the object and the film (object film distance) should be small as possible.
3. The object and film should be parallel to each other.

4. The source to object film distance should be as long as possible.

5. The central ray must strike the tooth, object and film at right angles.

6. There should be no movement of the tube, film or patient during exposure.

Q6. Define image sharpness.

Ans. It is the degree which defines how well a boundary between two differing radiodensities can be delineated. Image sharpness can be enhanced by; using small effective focal spot, increasing the distance between the focal spot and the object by using long cone, minimizing the distance between the object and the image receptor.

Q7. Define image resolution.

Ans. It is the degree which defines how well a radiograph records separate objects that are close together.

Q8. What are the causes of foreshortening and elongation of the image?

Ans. Foreshortening: When central ray is perpendicular to film but not to the object, the resultant image will be recorded shorter than its actual size, this type of dimensional distortion is called foreshortening of the image (applicable to paralleling technique).

Additionally; if excessive vertical angulation of central ray is used the resultant image will appear shorter than the actual size (applicable to bisecting angle technique).

Elongation: When central ray is perpendicular to the object but not to the film, the resultant image will be recorded elongated than its actual size, this type of distortion is called elongation of the image (applicable to paralleling technique).

If insufficient vertical angulation of central ray is used, the resultant image will appear elongated than the actual size (applicable to bisecting angle technique).

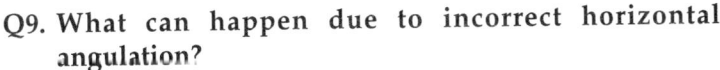

Q9. What can happen due to incorrect horizontal angulation?

Ans. If film and object are placed parallel to each other but central ray is not perpendicular to either of them, the geometric distortion will result in overlapping of adjacent anatomic structures.

Q10. What are the methods of object localization?

Ans. 1. Right angle technique
2. Tube shift technique or buccal object rule or Clark's rule
3. CT/CBCT.

Q11. What is right angle technique?

Ans. In this technique, occlusal view is taken with IOPA of the same region to localize object. These radiographs are right angle to each other in context with position of the central beam. In IOPA, if the object is appearing at apex of 36, occlusal view of the same region will give mediolateral position of that object.

Q12. What is tube shift technique or buccal object rule or Clark's rule?

Ans. This is also called SLOB, i.e. same lingual and opposite buccal. Two radiographs are taken at different angles to localize object. If the object appears to move in the same direction as the X-ray tube (suppose mesial) in second IOPA, it is on the lingual side. If it moves in opposite direction in relation to tube (tube moved mesially but object appeared distal to tooth), then object is on the buccal aspect. If object does not move with respect to the reference object (first IO PA), it denotes that the it lies at the same depth.

Q13. What is eggshell effect and how it occurs?

Ans. It is an appearance of corticated structures of the jaws on the radiographs as the image projected is a three-dimensional volume on a two-dimensional receptor. At the topmost point of egg (as at most expanded end of cortex), top photon has a tangential path and much longer path for lower photon through the shell of the egg as it travels through two thickness of the shell. So, photons travelling at periphery are more attenuated than photons travelling at right angles to the surface. The periphery of expanded cortex is more opaque than the region inside the expanded border.

X-Ray Films

X-ray Films, Intensifying Screens and Grids

Q1. What is composition of X-ray film?

Ans. **Emulsion:** Silver halide grains (silver iodide and silver bromide)

Base: Plastic supporting material.

Impurities like sulphur, silver, gold—to improve sensitivity of silver halide crystals.

Vehicle: Applied of both side of base—gelatinous and non-gelatinous material which keeps silver halide grains evenly dispersed.

Adhesive: For adhesion of emulsion to film base, a thin layer of adhesive is applied.

An additional layer of vehicle is added to the film emulsion as an overcoat; this barrier helps protect the film from damage by scratching, contamination, or pressure from rollers when an automatic processor is used.

Q2. What are direct exposure film?

Ans. Film intended to be exposed by X-rays is called direct exposure film.

Q3. What are screen films?

Ans. Screen film, which is sensitive to visible light, is used with intensifying screens that emit visible light. Screen film and intensifying screens are used for extraoral projections such as panoramic and skull radiographs.

Q4. What is function of base of X-ray film?

Ans. The function of the film base is to support the emulsion. The base must have the proper degree of flexibility to allow easy handling of the film. The base for dental X-ray film is 0.18 mm thick and is made of polyester polyethylene terephthalate. The film base is uniformly translucent and casts no pattern on the resultant radiograph. The film base must also withstand exposure to processing solutions without becoming distorted.

Q5. Why emulsion is applied on both sides of film?

Ans. With a double layer of emulsion, less radiation can be used to produce an image.

Q6. What are the uses of raised/embossed dot?

Ans. a. It helps in film orientation during X-ray taking
b. It is used to identify patient's side (Rt/Lt) after processing.

Q7. What is the function of black paper in X-ray film packet?

Ans. It protects the film from direct light.

Q8. What is the function of lead foil in X-ray film packet?

Ans. It is positioned behind the film and it shields the film from back scatter radiation or secondary radiation, thus improving image quality. To give rigidity to film. It also reduces patient's exposure.
if place reversed—tyre track pattern

Q9. What is the function of white or plastic wrapping?

Ans. If protects the film as it is resistant to moisture?

Q10. Enumerate image characteristics of X-ray film.

Ans. **Density:** The overall degree of darkening of an exposed film is referred to as radiographic density.

Contrast: Difference in densities between light and dark regions on a radiograph. Film contrast describes the capacity of radiographic films to display differences in subject contrast, that is, variations in the intensity of the remnant beam.

Radiographic speed: Radiographic speed refers to the amount of radiation required to produce an image of a standard density.

Film latitude: Film latitude is a measure of the range of exposures that can be recorded as distinguishable densities on a film.

Radiographic noise: Radiographic noise is the appearance of uneven density of a uniformly exposed radiographic film.

Resolution: Sharpness is the ability of a radiograph to define an edge precisely. Resolution, or resolving power, is the ability of a radiograph to record separate structures that are close together.

Film speed is also an important characteristic. It is a function of the number and size of the silver halide crystals in the emulsion. The larger the crystals, the faster is the film but poorer the image quality.

Q11. What is image receptor blurring?

Ans. With intraoral dental X-ray film, the size and number of the silver grains in the film emulsion determines image sharpness: the finer the grain size, the finer the sharpness. In general, slow–speed films have fine grains and faster films have larger grains.

Q12. What is motion blurring?

Ans. Image sharpness also can be lost through movement of the film, subject, or X-ray source during exposure. Movement of the X-ray source in effect enlarges the focal spot and diminishes image sharpness.

Q13. What is geometric blurring?

Ans. The larger the focal spot, the greater the loss of image sharpness causing blurring of resultant image.

Q14. What is parallax?

Ans. When wet films are viewed, the emulsion is swollen with water which causes loss of image sharpness, called parallax effect.

Q15. What is duplication?

Ans. Duplicating film has emulsion only on one side. In a dark room, this film is exposed to visible light in close contact with original film. This duplicate radiograph can be used patient for insurance claim and as reading aids.

Q16. Classify X-ray films.

Ans. i. Intraoral—IOPA, bitewing, occlusal.
Extraoral—OPG and other extraorals
ii. Screen film—with screen and non-screen films
iii. Speed—according to speed: A, B, C, D, E, F
iv. According to size—0, 1, 2, 3.
v. Emulsion—single emulsion, or double emulsion films.

Q17. Enlist sizes of films with dimensions.

Ans. Size 0, child (posterior)—22 × 35 mm
Size 1, child (anterior)—24 × 40 mm
Size 2, adult (posterior)—31 × 41 mm
Size 3, adult (anterior)—27 × 54 mm
Bitewing film = Size 2 film is used.
Occlusal film = 57 × 76 mm (size 4)

Q18. Set of full mouth radiographs consists of how many film.

Ans. Full mouth set: 6 anterior IOPA, 8 posterior IOPA and 4 bitewings (molar and premolar).

Q19. Type of film holders types are:

Ans. Blade type: Throat stick, acrylic blade with slot, Snap-A-ray
Bite block—Snap-A-ray, artery forceps with bite block
Positioning indicating device—Rinn XCP with collimator, precision X-ray holder

Q20. What are the advantages of film holder?

Ans. • Allows film to be placed parallel to long axis of teeth
• Helps to maintain flat planes
• Retaining the film in position till exposure

Q21. What are the disdavantages of film holder?

Ans. • It may not allow film to extend beyond apical region of teeth to cover more structures

• It can prevent operator from checking film position intraorally, once fixed in holder.

Q22. What is intensifying screen (IS)?

Ans. It is a device that transfers X-ray energy into visible light; the visible light in turn exposes the screen film. This method intensifies the effect of X-rays on the screen film with less amount of radiation to patient.

Advantage: Patient is exposed to less radiation

Disadvantage: Image unsharpness, need compatible screen film

Q23. Which are the rare earth materials used in IS?

Ans. Phosphorus (rare earth materials) used are terbium-activated gadolinium oxysulfide (TAGOS) emitting green light and niobium activated yttrium tantalate (NAYTL) emitting blue light and UV rays.

Q24. What is the composition of IS?

Ans. • Base—made of polyster plastic which gives mechanical support

• Phosphor coat—composed of phosphorescent crystals suspended in a polymeric binder. When the crystals absorb X-ray photons, they fluoresce.

• Protective layer—placed over phosphor coat to protect it and provide surface that can be cleaned.

Q25. What are grids?

Ans. Grids are used to prevent the scattered radiation from reaching the film. Scattered radiation causes fog and reduces contrast of the film.

Q26. What are the types of grids?

Ans. • Focused grids and non-focused grids

• Stationary grids and moving grids

Q27. What is the composition of grid?

Ans. It is composed of a series of long parallel strips of an opaque material usually lead, held apart and parallel to each other by an X-ray transparent interspace material like plastic.

Q28. What is the function of grid?

Ans. The grid is placed between the patient's head and the film. During exposure, the grid permits the passage of the X-ray beam between the lead strips. When X-rays interact with the patient's tissues, scattered radiation is produced; this scattering is directed at the grid and film at a particular angle. Due to this, scattered radiation are absorbed by the lead strips and does not reach the surface of the film to cause the film fog. Grid can remove 80–90% of scattering which helps to improve the contrast.

Q29. What is grid ratio?

Ans. The ratio between the height of the lead strip and the distance between them. The lead strip are 0.05 mm thick. Interspaces are much thicker than the lead strips. Grid ratio usually ranges from 4:1 to 16:1.

Q30. What are the advantages of grids?

Ans. 1. Reduces film fog and increases radiographic contrast.
   2. Grid can be used to aid in the measurement of relative bone height with the help of radiographs.

Q31. What is the disadvantage of grids?

Ans. It needs double amount of exposure compared to radiographs taken in absence of grids.

   Note: Grid should be used only when improved image quality and high contrast are necessary.

Processing

Q1. Enlist dark room equipment.

Ans. • Safelight (low intensity) with long wave length
   • Processing tanks
   • Thermometer
   • Drying racks
   • Timer

Q2. What are the specifications for safe light?

Ans. Safelight should be of low intensity and long wavelength, which should not affect the film but can allow one to visualize the area in the dark room. It should be mounted on the wall 4 feet away from the work area using red GBX-2 filter and frosted 15 watt bulb.

Q3. Enlist the steps of film processing.

Ans. • Immerse exposed film in developer—20 seconds (depending on the concentration of solution)
   • Rinse in water to wash out developer—30 seconds
   • Immerse in the fixer—8–10 minutes
   • Rinse in water to wash out fixer—1 minute.
   • Dry and mount the film—till no water drop exist and emulsion dries completely.

Q4.

	Contents	Action
Developer	Phenidone, hydroquinone	Converts exposed silver halide crystals into metallic silver
Activator	Sodium or potassium hydroxide	Maintains the pH of solution and cause gelatin to swell to allow developing agent to diffuse rapidly into emulsion
Preservative	Antioxidant – sodium sulfite	Increases the shelf life of solution
Restrainer	Bromide containing KBr compounds	Antifog agent

Q5.

Fixer	Contents	Action
Clearing agent	Ammonium thiosulfate	Dissolves the unexposed silver halide grains
Acidifier	Acetic acid	Allows diffusion of thiosulfate into emulsion and inactivates residual developing agent by acidic pH
Preservative	Ammonium sulfite	Prevents oxidation of thio-sulfate
Hardener	Aluminium sulfate	Complexes with gelatin and prevents damage to film while handling, also reduces swelling of emulsion to shorten the drying time

Q6. What are the different methods of processing?

Ans. They are:

a. Manual method which includes time temperature method and visual method

b. Automatic method (automatic processor)

c. Monobath

d. Self developing films

e. Day light method

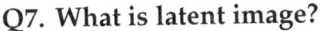

Q7. What is latent image?

Ans. When the dental radiographic film is exposed to X-rays, the silver halide crystals interact with photons and get chemically changed. These chemically altered crystals are said to constitute the latent image.

Q8. How is latent image formed?

Ans. Silver halide crystals have interstitial silver ions in crystal lattice as imperfections. Sulfur compounds added to film sensitize silver halide crystals causing irregularities in the crystal. These areas are called latent image sites. These sites function when electrons are trapped in them after the film/emulsion is irradiated. Processing solutions converts the crystals with latent image into black metallic silver grains that can be visualized and removes the unexposed silver bromide crystals.

Errors	Light radiograph	Dark radiograph	Insufficient contrast	Film fog (dark film)	Dark spots or lines	Light spots	Yellow/Brown stains	Blurring
C	Under development	Over development	Under development	Improper safelight	Finger-print contamination	Film contaminated with fixer before processing	Depleted developer	Movement of patient
A	Excessive fixation	Under fixation	Under exposure	Light leaks	Film in contact with tank	Film in contact with tank	Depleted fixer	Movement of X-ray tube head
U	Under exposure (low kVp, mA, time)	Improper safelight	Excessive kVp	Over development	Excessive bending of film	Excessive bending of film	Insufficient washing	Double exposure
S	Film source distance too great	Over exposure	Excessive film fog	Contaminated solutions	Film contact with developer before processing	Film contact with fixer before processing	Contaminated solutions	
E	Film packet reversed in mouth	Film source distance too short		Deteriorated film				

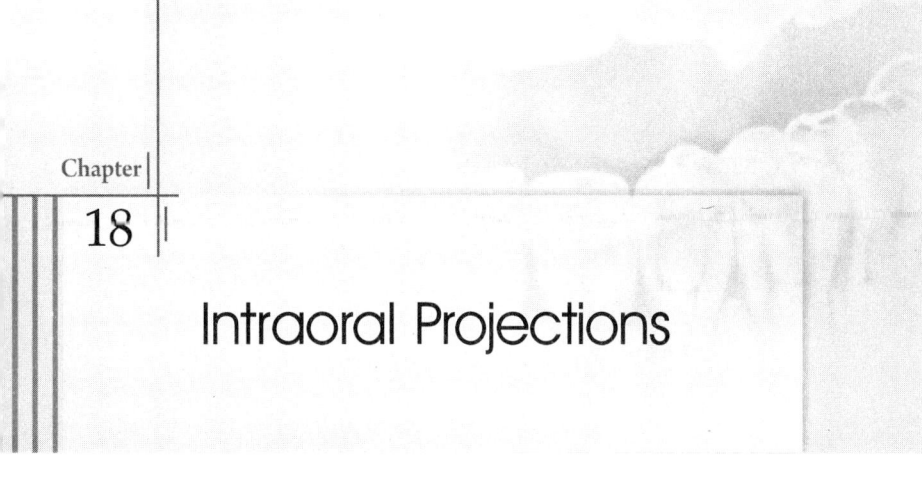

Intraoral Projections

Q1. What are the advantages of long cone technique or paralleling technique?

Ans. 1. Accuracy: The image produce is geometrically accurate. The image is free of distortion and exhibits detail and definition. There is no overlap of structures.

2. The technique is simple and easy to learn and use

3. Technique is easy to standardize and can be accurately duplicated or repeated, when serial radiographs are indicated.

4. The radiographs produced give; an excellent bone level assessment, clear involvement by interproximal caries and images without elongation and fore-shortening.

5. Useful in handicapped and compromised patients.

Q2. What are the disadvantages of long cone technique or paralleling technique?

Ans. 1. Film placement is difficult in child patients and adults with small mouth or shallow palate.

2. The film holding device may impinge on the oral soft tissues and cause discomfort and gagging

3. Object film distance is more so more exposure.

4. Positioning in third molar region is difficult

5. The film holders need to be autoclavable.

Q3. What are the disadvantages bisecting angle technique?

Ans. 1. Patient's hand is in the path of the primary beam, thus leading to unnecessary exposure

2. Patient may use excessive force to stabilize the film causing bending of the film which can cause image distortion

3. Patient may allow the film to slip from its position resulting in inadequate exposure of the prescribed area

4. More chances of operator error such as cone cut and image distortion.

Q4. What are the advantages bisecting angle technique?

Ans. 1. Positioning of image receptor is reasonably comfortable for the patient in all areas of mouth

2. Positioning is relatively simple and quick.

3. If all angulations are assessed correctly, the image of the tooth will be same length as the tooth itself and should be adequate (but not ideal) for most diagnostic purposes.

Q5. What are the indications of occlusal radiography?

Ans. 1. To precisely locate roots and supernumerary, unerupted and impacted teeth.

2. To localize foreign bodies in the jaws and stones in the ducts of sublingual and submandibular glands.

3. To demonstrate and evaluate the integrity of the anterior, medial and lateral outlines of the maxillary sinus.

4. To aid in the examination of patients with trismus.

5. To obtain information about the location, nature, extent and displacement of fractures of the mandible and maxilla.

6. To determine the medial and lateral extent of the disease (cyst, osteomyelitis, malignancy).

7. To detect disease in the palate or floor of the mouth.

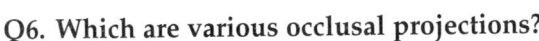

Q6. Which are various occlusal projections?

Ans. *For maxillary arch*

- Anterior maxillary occlusal projection
- Cross-sectional maxillary occlusal projection
- Lateral maxillary occlusal projection

For mandibular arch

- Anterior mandibular occlusal projection
- Cross-sectional mandibular occlusal projection
- Lateral mandibular occlusal projection

Q7. Which are the indications of bitewing radiography?

Ans. 1. Detection of initial dental caries at the proximal surface and at the occlusal D-E junction.

2. Detection of secondary dental caries especially at the pulpal and cervical floor.

3. To study proximity of carious lesion to pulp

4. Detection of early periodontal disease

5. Also effective in detection of interproximal calculus.

Q8. Which are two bitewing projections?

Ans. 1. Premolar bitewing projection

2. Molar bitewing projection.

Intraoral Anatomy

Q1. **Enumerate maxillary and mandibular anatomic landmarks.**

Or

List four radiopaque landmarks of maxilla.

List four radiopaque landmarks of mandible.

List four radiolucent landmarks of maxilla.

List four radiolucent landmarks of maxilla.

Ans.

	Maxilla	Mandible	Common Landmarks
Radio-lucent (RL)	• Intermaxillary suture • Nasal aperture • Incisive foramen • Superior foramina of the nasopalatine canal • Lateral fossa • Nasolacrimal canal • Maxillary sinus	• Symphysis (at early age) • Lingual foramen • Mental fossa • Mental foramen • Mandibular canal • Nutrient canal • Submandibular gland fossa	Lamina dura, developing tooth crypt—RO

Contd.

Contd.

	Maxilla	*Mandible*	*Common Landmarks*
Radio-opaque (RO)	• Anterior nasal spine • Nose • Zygomatic process and zygoma • Nasolabial fold • Pterygoid plates	• Genial tubercles • Mental ridge • Mylohyoid ridge • External oblique ridge • Inferior border of mandible • Coronoid process	Alveolar crest—RO Pulp chamber/canal, PDLS, nutrient canal—RL Cancellous bone—RO + RL

Q2. Which anatomic structure of mandible can be seen in maxillary posterior IOPA radiographs?

Ans. Coronoid process

Q3. What is Y line of ennis?

Ans. It is radiopaque structure formed by intersection of maxillary sinus and the nasal cavity.

Q4. Which are other soft tissue structures which appear radiopaque on the radiographs?

Ans. • Soft tissue of nose seen usually with maxillary incisors.
• Nasolabial fold appear as oblique line at maxillary premolar region

Q5. Nutrient canals are prominent in which disorder?

Ans. Nutrient canals are commonly seen as prominent structure in patients with hypertension.

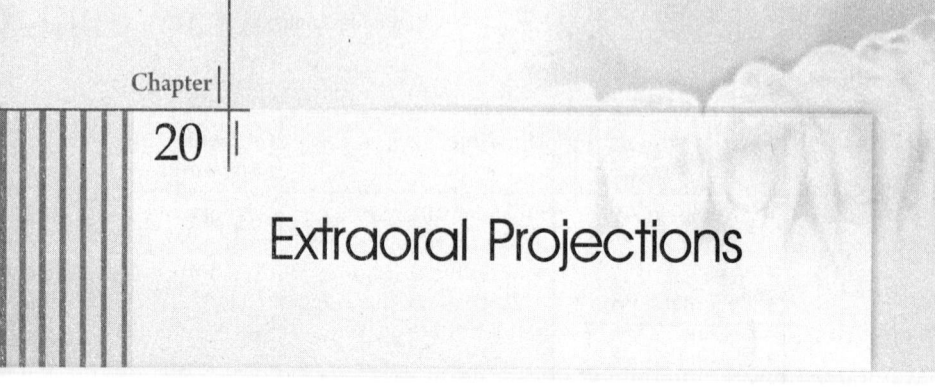

Extraoral Projections

Extraoral Radiography

Q1. What are the main indications for skull and maxillo-facial radiography?

Ans. a. Fractures of the maxillofacial skeleton
b. Fractures of the skull
c. Investigation of the antra (sinuses)
d. Diseases affecting the skull base and vault
e. TMJ disorders.

Q2. What are the main indications of lateral oblique radiographs? (Body/Ramus)

Ans. a. Assessment of presence and or position of unerupted teeth in body or ramus.
b. Detection of fracture of mandible
c. Evaluation of lesions or conditions affecting jaws
d. As an alternative to intraoral view
e. Salivary gland and TMJ pathology analysis.

Q3. What is bimolar technique/Gardner's view?

Ans. Bimolar is term used for the radiographic projection showing oblique lateral views of the right and left sides of the jaws on the different halves of the same radiographs.

Q4. What are the main indications for lateral cephalogram?

Ans. For orthodontic evaluation and to visualise
• Sphenoid sinus
• Frontal sinus

- Nasal bones
- Maxillary sinus
- Orbit
- Anterior maxilla and mandible

Q5. What are the main indications for submentovertex view?

Ans. To visualise
- **Zygomatic arch**
- Sphenoid sinus
- Ethmoid sinus
- Condylar head
- Posterior maxilla
- Anterior mandible

Q6. What is jug handle view and its indication?

Ans. Jug handle view is modified submentovertex projection with lesser exposure to visualize fractures of zygomatic arch.

Q7. Which are the main indications for water's projection?

Ans. To visualise
- **Maxillary sinus**
- Coronoid process
- Orbit zygoma
- **Ethmoid sinus**
- **Frontal sinus**
- Zygomatic arch
- Nasal bones.

Q8. What are the main indications for PA ceph view?

Ans. To visualise
- Orbit
- Nasal cavity
- Frontal sinus
- Anterior maxilla

- Ramus
- Mandibular body
- Coronoid process
- Condylar neck.

Q9. What are the main indications of reverse Towne view?

Ans. To visualise

- Condylar neck—bilateral fractures of condyle and displacement
- Condylar head

Q10. Which are the main indications of panoramic view?

Ans. To visualise

- Mandibular body
- Ramus
- Posterior maxilla
- Coronoid process
- Condylar neck
- Anterior maxilla
- Zygoma
- Frontal sinus.

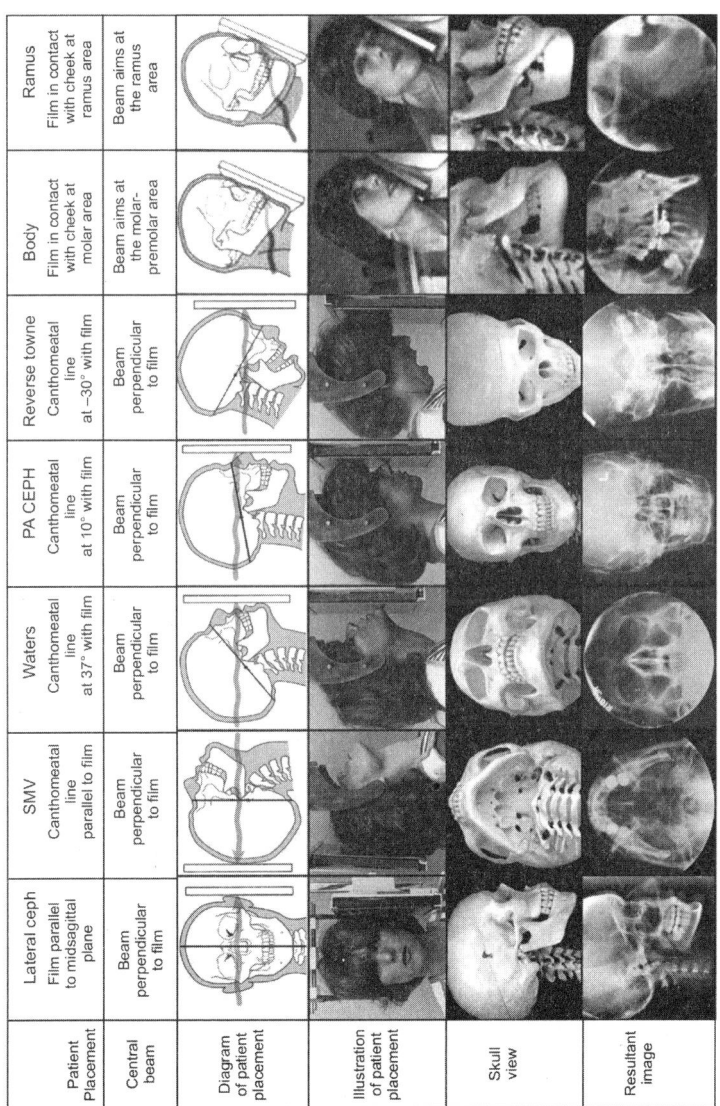

Various projections of extraoral radiography (white and pharoah)

	Lateral ceph	SMV	Waters	PA CEPH	Reverse towne	Body	Ramus
Patient Placement	Film parallel to midsagittal plane	Canthomeatal line parallel to film	Canthomeatal line at 37° with film	Canthomeatal line at 10° with film	Canthomeatal line at −30° with film	Film in contact with cheek at molar area	Film in contact with cheek at ramus area
Central beam	Beam perpendicular to film	Beam perpendicular to film	Beam perpendicular to film	Beam perpendicular to film	Beam perpendicular to film	Beam aims at the molar-premolar area	Beam aims at the ramus area
Diagram of patient placement							
Illustration of patient placement							
Skull view							
Resultant image							

Panoramic Imaging

Panoramic Radiography

Q1. What is the principle of OPG functioning?

Ans. OPG works on the principle of **tomography** and **slit beam collimation**. If the film moves with the same speed at one particular point or object, this point will always be projected on the same spot on the film and not appear unsharp. In panoramic radiography the film is attached to a rotating system and moves in the opposite direction to the beam. The film and X-ray beam are given the correct speed to rotate in opposing direction to produce an image on the object given.

Q2. What is focal trough or image layer?

Ans. It is a three-dimensional imaginary curved zone in which structures lying within are clearly demonstrated on a panoramic radiograph. It is the zone which contains those object or points which are depicted with optimum resolution.

Q3. What are the indications of OPG?

Ans. • As a substitute for full mouth intraoral periapical radiographs.
• For evaluation of tooth development for children, the mixed dentition and also the age.
• To assist and assess the patient for and during orthodontic treatment.
• To establish the site and size of lesions such as cysts, tumors and developmental anomalies in the body and rami of the mandible.

- Prior to any surgical procedures such as extraction of impacted teeth, enucleation of a cyst, etc.
- For detection of fractures of the middle third face and the mandible after facial trauma.
- For follow-up of treatment, progress of pathology or postoperative bony healing.
- Investigation of TM joint dysfunction.
- To study the antrum, especially to study the floor, posterior and anterior walls of the antrum.
- Periodontal disease—as an overall view of the alveolar bone levels.
- Assessment for underlying bone disease before constructing complete or partial dentures.
- Evaluation of developmental anomalies.
- Implants

Q4. What are the advantages of OPG?

Ans.
- Simple procedure requiring very little patient compliance.
- Convenient for the patient.
- Useful in patients with trismus and gagging problems.
- Time required is minimal compared to a full mouth intraoral periapical radiographs.
- That portion of the maxilla and the mandible lying within the focal trough can be visualized on a single film.
- The patient dose is relatively low as compared to full mouth X-rays.
- Panoramic radiographs taken for diagnostic purpose are valuable visual aid in patient education.
- Useful for mass screening.

Q5. What are the disadvantages of OPG?

Ans.
- Areas of diagnostic interest outside the focal trough may be poorly visualized, e.g. swelling on the palate, floor of the mouth.
  - Comparatively this radiograph is of a poor diagnostic quality, in terms of **magnification**, geometric **distortion,** poor definition and **loss of detail** an sharpness.

- There is an *overlapping* of the teeth in the bicuspid area of the maxilla and the mandible.
- Number of radiopaque and radiolucent areas may be present due to the superimposition of real/double or *ghost images* and because of *soft tissue shadows* and *airspaces*.

Q6. Errors, their causes and radiographic appearences.

Sr. No.	Errors	Reason	Radiographic appearance
a.	Ghost image	Produced when a radiodense object is penetrated twice by the X-ray beam.	**Failure to remove necklace**
			Failure to remove ear-rings
b.	Lead apron artifact	When lead apron comes in exposure or by wearing it too high.	
c.	Reverse smile appearance	Chin is positioned too high or tipped up	
d.	Exaggerated smile appearance • Shortening of lower incisors	Chin is positioned too low	

Contd.

Contd.

Sr. No.	Errors	Reason	Radiographic appearance
e.	Patient positioned too forward on bite block	Anterior teeth appear narrow	
f.	Patient is positioned too far back on the bite block	Anterior teeth appear widened and blurred	
g.	Patient head tilted to one side	The side tilted towards the X-ray tube is enlarged	
h.	Positioning of the spine	If the patient is not sitting or standing with a straight spine, the cervical spine appears as a pyramid-shaped radiopacity in the centre of the film and obscures diagnostic information. (arrows indicating tongue shadow)	
i.	Continuous shaking movement throughout the cycle	Due to movement of patient during exposure, image appears blurred	

Digital Imaging

Q1. What are the methods by which intraoral digital image can be obtained?

Ans. **Direct digital imaging:** A sensor is placed at the area of interest like an IOPA film and exposed to radiation. After X-ray exposure, the sensor captures the radiographic image and then it is transferred to computer.

Indirect digital imaging: In this method an existing X-ray film is digitized using a CCD camera and then displayed on the computer monitor.

Storage phosphor imaging: A reusable imaging plate coated with phosphor is used. These PSP (photostimulable phosphor plate) plates are flexible and fit into the mouth. The storage phosphor imaging records diagnostic data on the plates following exposure to the X-ray source and uses a high-speed scanner to convert the information to electronic files which can be displayed on the computer screen.

Q2. By which method extraoral digital image can be obtained?

Ans. Storage phosphor imaging (PSP) and indirect digital imaging (CCD) methods are used for extraoral images.

Q3. What are the different types of sensor or digital detecters?

Ans. Charged couple device (CCD)
   • Complementary metal oxide semiconductors (CMOS)

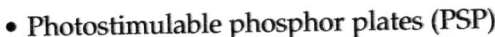

- Photostimulable phosphor plates (PSP)
- Flat panel detectors

Q4. Advantages of digital imaging.

Ans. 1. Superior gray scale resolution

2. Reduced exposure to radiation

3. **Faster image viewing**

4. No need of film/dark room/processing solution

5. Excellent quality image with no loss of quality

6. Image manipulation for specific diagnostic purpose is possible

7. Effective patient education tool.

8. Easy to store

Q5. Disadvantages of digital imaging.

Ans. 1. Costly equipment

2. Image manipulation can be unethical

3. Sensor size is thicker than intraoral films and therefore lacks patient compliance

4. Infection control is mandatory

5. It is debatable whether digital radiographs can be used as evidence in lawsuits.

Q6. What are the common problems in digital imaging receptors related to exposure, processing and handling?

Ans. • There can be radiographic noise.

- PSP plate exposure to excessive light before exposure can lead to non-uniform image density.

- Bending of sensor/plate may give distorted image

- Incomplete erasure of sensors can show double images

- Damaged or overused plates/sensors can direct towards unnecessary retake of image.

Q7. Difference between film imaging and digital imaging.

Ans.

	Film imaging	Digital imaging
1.	No need of receptor preparation	Receptor preparation is needed
2.	Film can be placed with the help of holders and can be placed to approximate anatomy	Inflexible receptors and bulky so difficult patient compliance, cannot be placed as per anatomic variations.
3.	Needs time to visualize image	Immediate display on computer with CCD/CMOS
4.	Any light source gives quick image evaluation	Needs set up of processor and monitor
5.	Duplicated image is inferior to original	Electronic copies can be stored without loss of image quality

Cone Beam Computed Tomography (CBCT)

Q1. What are the other names for CBCT?

Ans. DVT—digital volumetric tomography

VT—volumetric tomography

Q2. Why is CBCT named so?

Ans. This technology is base on the principle of tomography (tomo = slices), and the shape of the X-ray beam used for imaging is cone-shaped hence it is named as cone beam computed tomography.

Q 3. What is field of view?

Ans. It is an area which is covered during scanning anatomical region as required. It varies according to manufacturer to ensure limited dose delivery to jaws.

Q4. Field of view (FOV) depends on which factors?

Ans. • The dimensions of the FOV or scan volume generated depend principally on:

• The detector size and shape

• The beam projection geometry

• Collimation of the beam.

Q5. Which are commonly used dimensions of FOV?

Ans. Small = 5 × 5 cm

Medium = 10 × 10 /8 × 8 cm

Large = 17 × 11

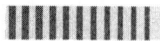

Q6. What are the advantages of CBCT over conventional radiography?

Ans. CBCT exhibits various advantages over conventional radiographic techniques, minimal magnification, no geometric distortion, and appropriate multiplanar and 3D displays. This technology ensures improved structure visualization and diagnostic efficacy.

Q7. What are the limitations of CBCT imaging?

Ans. 1. High cost of the equipment and imaging studies

2. Higher radiation dose as compared to conventional radiographs

3. Requires skilled and experienced personnel for generation and interpretation of the resultant data.

4. Prolonged time required for image manipulation and interpretation.

5. Artifacts in the image.

Q8. What are the various clinical applications of CBCT?

Ans. • *Prosthodntics:* **Implant planning** and anatomical considerations: Planning of precise implant position

• *Maxillofacial surgery:* The evaluation of impacted teeth, supernumerary, unerupted teeth and their relation to vital structures.

• Obstructive sleep apnea.

• *Periodontics:* **Measurements of intra-bony defects** dehiscence, fenestration defects and periodontal pathologies.

• *Endodontics:* Root morphology-shape, location, number of canals missed canals.

• Orthodontia: Orthodontic assessment and cephalomatric analysis

• *TMJ:* To delineate the true position of the condyle in the fossa.

• Oropharyngeal volume

• Forensic dentistry

• ENT.

Q9. Enlist five differences between CT and CBCT.

Ans.

S No	CT	CBCT
1.	Operates at a higher voltage than CBCT	Operating voltage same as OPG, 80–120 kVp
2.	Rotating anode	Stationary anode
3.	High radiation dose to patient	Pulsed X-ray beam generation so less radiation dose to patient
4.	Beam rotates at 360° during exposure	Cone-shaped beam
5.	HU: Used to express CT numbers in standardized form as per tissue density it varies	Gray values: Not standardized to measure tissue density as HU in CT

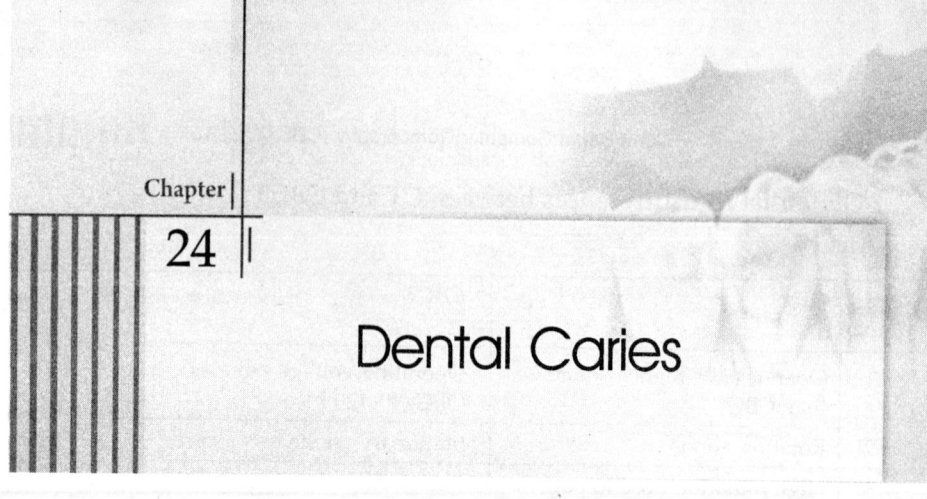

Dental Caries

Q1. Classify caries according to radiographic appearance.

Ans. A. According to the severity and extent of the lesion: Incipient, moderate, advanced, severe.

    B. According to the location on the tooth:
Pit and fissure caries
- Occlusal
- Buccal/Lingual pit.

Smooth surface caries
- Proximal
- Buccal or lingual surfaces
- Root surface caries.

Recurrent caries

    C. According to etiology
- Recurrent caries
- Rampant caries
- Radiation caries.

Q2. Which are the radiographic techniques used to detect caries.

Ans. IOPA: It helps to detect gross carious lesions, root surface caries and changes in the apical and inter-radicular bone due to caries.

Bitewing: It helps to detect caries in interproximal areas and distal ends of premolars and molars, and caries at CE junction.

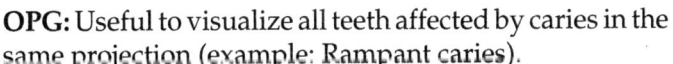

OPG: Useful to visualize all teeth affected by caries in the same projection (example: Rampant caries).

Q3. Give differential diagnosis of dental caries.

Ans. Cervical burn out: Located at the neck of the teeth, triangular in shape, gradually becoming less apparent towards the centre of the tooth, follows anatomical contour and the peripheral border appears intact. Many teeth in the same arch on the radiograph will appear to be affected.

Internal resorption: Enlarged pulp chamber. The margins are sharp and smooth. Lesion can be symmetric or eccentric.

External resorption: Seen at apices of teeth, blunt apex, smooth outline altering shape of root.

Erosion cavity: Saucer-shaped radiolucency with well defined or diffuse borders.

Nonopaque filling: It will have sharpness and uniformity of the margins.

Hypoplasia of enamel: Several small dark spots are seen in multiple teeth.

   Irregular attrition or abrasion can also be included as DD of caries.

Q4. What are the limitation of 2D radiographic technique to detect caries?

Ans. Standardization of technique is necessary to get similar view, as it is 2D image of three-dimensional structure. **Technique variation** in vertical tube head position may cause recurrent carious lesions to be obscured. **Exposure factors** can also affect the appearance or size of carious lesions.

Periodontal Diseases

Q1. Which periodontal changes can be diagnosed with the help of radiographs?

Ans.
- Condition of the alveolar crests
- Bone loss in furcation areas
- Width of the periodontal ligament space other factors affecting periodontium can also be visualized, like calculus, poorly contoured or over extended restorations, root length and morphology and the crown to root ratio.

Q.2. What are the limitations of 2D radiograph in diagnosing periodontal diseases?

Ans.
- It is difficult to differentiate between the buccal and lingual crestal bone levels.
- Only part of a complex bony defect is shown.
- One wall of a bone defect may obscure the rest of the defect.
- Bone resorption in the furcation area may be obscured by an overlying root or bone shadow.
- Early (incipient) destructive lesion in the bone are not detected on the radiograph.

Q3. Which are the common radiographs used to detect periodontal disease?

Ans.
- The **bitewing** and **periapical radiographs** are useful for evaluating the periodontium. *Intraoral grids* may be supplemented to evaluate the bone height.

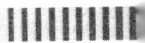

- **Digital subtraction radiography** including subtraction radiography and densitometric image analysis
- In **CBCT**, the axial, coronal and sagittal sections obtained help to evaluate the extent of bone loss.
- Clinicians also use **OPG** for initial screening of the jaws affected by periodontitis.

Q4. Which are the systemic condition affecting the periodontium?

Ans. • Pregnancy
- Uncontrolled diabetes
- Drugs, e.g. nifedipine
- HIV
- Leukemia
- Down's syndrome
- Langerhans' cell disease (histiocytosis X)
- Papillon-Lefevre syndrome
- Secondary metastases.

Q5. Periodontal conditions with radiographic features:

Ans. a. Early or mild periodontitis—an area of localized erosion of the alveolar bone crest.

b. Moderate periodontitis—when the destruction of the alveolar bone extends beyond the early changes on the alveolar crest and may induce variety of defects. The buccal and lingual cortical plate can get resorbed.

c. Horizontal bone loss—loss of height of the alveolar bone with the crest still horizontal or parallel to the occlusal plane which is classified into mild, moderate or severe depending upon the extent.

d. Vertical osseous defects—vertical (angular) bony lesions that are localized to one or two teeth. They are difficult to diagnose on a radiograph because one or both of the cortical bony plates can get superimposed with the defect.

e. Advance or severe periodontitis—extensive bone loss with excessive mobility and drifting of the remaining

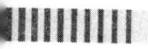

teeth. This may be accompanied with extensive horizontal bone loss or extensive osseous defects.

Q6. Give differential diagnosis of periodontal disease.

Ans. • Periodontal disease should be differentiated from following conditions with clinical co-relation:

- Squamous cell carcinoma, which usually shows extensive localized destruction of bone, with invasive tendency

- *Langerhans' cell histiocytosis (eosinophilic granuloma):* Usually no particular tooth is targeted and the midroot region is the epicenter of bone destruction which gives the lesion an ice cream scoop appearance. The alveolar crest remains intact.

- *Effect of systemic diseases on periodontal disease:* Few diseases which appear to influence the periodontium and periodontal treatments are: Diabetes mellitus, hematologic disorders, genetic and hereditary disturbances, hormonal changes and stress. Diabetes mellitus patients show severe and rapid alveolar bone resorption and are prone to develop periodontal abscesses.

- *AIDS:* There is rapid progression that leads to bone sequestration and loss of multiple teeth.

Periapical Pathologies

S. No.	Pathology	Clinical features	Radiographic features
1.	Acute apical periodontitis	Nonvital tooth Sensitivity +/- Tender on percussion	Widening of PDLS
2.	Acute periapical abscess	Nonvital tooth Sensitivity +/- Tender on percussion Fever+ Lymphadenopathy+ Swelling +/-	Slight widening of the PDLs rarefaction unsharpness of the trabeculae, periapical ill defined radiolucency Loss of lamina dura.
4.	Chronic apical periodontitis	Usually asymptomatic	May show dense trabeculae as a sign of chronicity
5.	Chronic alveolar abscess	History of pain from dull to severe Nonvital tooth Sinus may be present Lymphadenopathy+	Ill defined radiolucent lesion with loss of lamina dura
6.	Periapical granuloma	Asymptomatic Discolored tooth . Involved tooth may show a deep restoration, extensive caries, fracture or	Well defined radioluceny without sclerotic border less than 1.5 cm in diameter

(Contd.)

(Contd.)

S. No.	Pathology	Clinical features	Radiographic features
		narrow pulp canal with nonvital pulp.	
7.	Periapical cyst	Bony hard swelling Crepitations+ Thinned out cortical bone giving rubbery consistency on palpation Long standing Carious affected tooth nonvital tooth	Round or pear shaped periapical radiolucency with hyperostotic borders more than 1.5 cm (but less than 3 cm) Displaced adjacent teeth Expansion of cortices
8	Periapical scar	H/o RCT or root resection	Well defined radiolucency smaller than granuloma Size is constant
9	Condensing osteitis	Nonvital tooth Long standing asymptomatic carious tooth	Thickened trabeculae can be seen in continuation with normal adjacent trabecuale The changes take place outside lamina dura. Periapical radiolucency surrounded by radio-opacity.
10	Osteosclerosis	No associated signs or symtoms Vital tooth	Solitary multiple roughly round radiopacity Occur around roots of teeth subjected to high occlusal forces

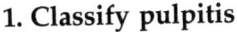

1. Classify pulpitis
  1. Pulpitis: Inflammatory disease of dental pulp.
     a. Reversible pulpitis:
        • Symptomatic (acute).
        • Asymptomatic (chronic).
     b. Irreversible pulpitis:
        • Acute
           – Abnormally responsive to cold, or
           – Abnormally responsive to heat.
        • Chronic
           – Asymptomatic with pulp exposure.
           – Hyperplastic pulpitis.
           – Internal resorption.
  2. Pulp degeneration:
     a. Calcific (radiographic diagnosis).
     b. Other (histopathological diagnosis).
  3. Pulp necrosis:
     a. Coagulation necrosis.
     b. Lique faction necrosis.
2. Radiographic features of osteomyelitis
  • **Acute suppurative osteomyelitis:** No radiographic changes observed. Radiographic changes can be observed only after about 10 days after the initiation of an acute bone infection, after structural alterations have occurred. The density of the involved bone is decreased and loss of sharpness of the trabeculae, outline becomes blurred or fuzzy.
  • **Osteomyelitis in infants:** No changes are seen for at least three weeks, after which irregular demineralization and other changes as those seen in acute osteomyelitis may be observed.
  • **Chronic, secondary type of suppurative osteomyelitis:** Multiple radiolucencies of variable size with irregular outline and poorly defined borders are seen the bone gradually develops 'a moth-eaten' appearance, as

radiolucent areas enlarge and are separated by islands of normal bone. Segaments of the necrotic bone become detached and calcified are called '*sequestra*'.

- **Sclerosing osteomyelitis:** There is a well circumscribed radiopaque apical mass often mimicking benign cementoblastoma. The root outline is always visible on the radiograph.

- **Diffuse sclerosing osteomyelitis:** Stripped or granular densification of bone, caused by subperiosteal deposition of new bone, obscures the intrinsic bone structure or deposition of new bone on the surface of marrow spaces. The deposition is more on the buccal and inferior surface of the jaw. Shortening of the roots of the involved teeth is seen.

- **Garre's osteomyelitis (proliferative periostitis):** An intraoral periapical radiograph will show a carious tooth opposite the hard bony mass. As infection persists the cortex thickens and becomes *laminated* with alternating radiopaque—radiolucent layers **(onion peel appearance)** Adjacent cancellous bone may remain normal, become sclerotic or show some areas of steolytic changes within the scleroses spongiosa. Following removal of the irritation, the cortical bone may remodel to a normal appearance.

Cysts of the Jaws

Table 16.1: Classification of cysts

Odontogenic cyst	Non odonto-genic cyst	Cyst of soft tissue origin	False cyst/cyst like lesion
Radicular cyst	Nasopalatine duct cyst	Thyroglossal duct cyst	Solitary/simple bone cyst
Residual cyst	Nasolabial cyst	Lymphoepithelial cyst of parotid	Stafne's cyst
Dentigerous cyst		Dermoid cyst	
Buccal bifurcation cyst		Branchial cleft cyst	
Keratocystic odontogenic tumor			
Glandular odontogenic cyst			
Calcified cystic odontogenic tumor			

Q1. Define cyst?

Ans. A cyst is a pathologic cavity filled with fluid, semiliquid or gaseous material which may or may not be lined by epithelium, and surrounded by a defined connective tissue wall.

Q2. What is the radiological appearance of periapical (radicular) cyst?

Ans. Round-shaped well-defined R/L with corticated border located at apex of a non-vital tooth.

Q3. How will you differntiate a radicular cyst from an apical granuloma?

Ans. • Radicular cyst has well-defined corticated hyperostotic borders

• A lesion of size more than 1.5 mm is more likely to be radicular cyst.

• Clinically granuloma is asymptomatic where as cyst may show eggshell crackling, swelling, mobility of teeth, and fluctuation

Q4. What is the radiological appearance of dentigerous cyst?

Ans. Well-defined R/L surrounding crown of involved tooth with cyst lining attacted at its CEJ.

Q5. How will you classify dentigerous cyst based on its radiological appearance?

Ans. • Central type

• Lateral type

• Circumferential type

Q6. What is the effect of dentigerous cyst on surrounding structure?

Ans. It *displaces* the associated tooth in apical direction. Degree of displacement may be considerable. It commonly displace the associated tooth in an apical direction.

Q7. How will you differentiate between a dentigerous cyst and normal follicular space radiologically?

Ans. The size of the normal follicular space is 2 to 3 mm. If the follicular space exceeds 5 mm, a dentigerous cyst is more likely.

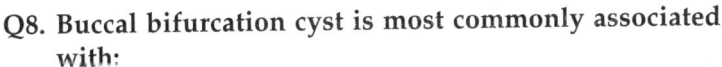

Q8. Buccal bifurcation cyst is most commonly associated with:

Ans. Mandibular first molar followed by the second molar.

Q9. Diagnostic characteristic of buccal furcation cyst is:

Ans. Tipping of the involved molar so that the root tips are pushed into the lingual cortical plate of the mandible and the occlusal surface is tipped toward the buccal aspect of the mandible.

Q10. Best diagnostic film for abnormally positioned roots in BBC is:

Ans. The best diagnostic film is the cross-sectional (standard) mandibular occlusal projection, which demonstrates the abnormal position of the tooth roots.

Q11. Most common location of KOT is:

Ans. The most common location of KOTs is the posterior body of the mandible (90% occur posterior to the canines) and ramus (>50%)

Q12. What is the effect of growing KOT on jaw?

Ans. Grow along the internal aspect of the jaws, causing minimal expansion of the cortical plates.

Q13. How will you give differential diagnosis between KOT and ameloblastoma?

Ans. The typical scalloped margin and multilocular appearance of the KOT may resemble an ameloblastoma, but the latter has a greater propensity to expand bucco-lingually.

Q14. What is the radiological appearance of skull in basal cell nevus syndrome?

Ans. Radiopaque line of the calcified falx cerebri may be prominent on the posteroanterior skull projection.

Q15. Lateral periodontal cyst are commonly located in:

Ans. 50% to 75% develop in the mandible, mostly in a region extending from the lateral incisor to the second premolar.

Q16. What is the common location of calcifying epithelial odontogenic cyst?

Ans. Most (75%) occurs in premolar/molar region, especially associated with cuspids and incisors.

Q17. What is the radiological appearance of CEOC?

Ans. Completely R/L or small foci of calcified material appearing as white flakes or small smooth pebbles. Completely radiolucent; it may show evidence of small foci of calcified material that appear as white flecks or small smooth pebbles.

Q18. How will you give differential diagnosis between median palatal cyst and nosopalatine duct cyst?

Ans. Most nasopalatine duct cysts are found in the nosopalatine foramen or canal. However, if this cyst extends posteriorly to involve the hard palate it often is referred to as a median palatal cyst.

Q19. What is the characteristic appearance of nasopalatine dust cyst?

Or

What is the reason for heart-shaped appearance of nosopalatine duct cyst?

Ans. The shadow of the nasal spine sometimes is superimposed on the cyst, giving it a heart shape.

Q20. How will you give differential diagnosis of incisive foramen and nanopalatine duct cyst?

Ans. Foramen larger than 6 mm may appear like a cysts it can be differentiated as:
- Displacement of teeth seen
- History
- Aspiration

Q21. What are the imaging modalities used for diagnosis of nasolabial cyst?

Ans. The investigation could include either CT imaging or magnetic resonance imaging, both of which can provide an image of soft tissues.

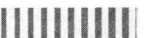

Q22. What is the common location of simple bone cyst?

Ans. Almost all SBCs are found in the mandible, in rare cases they develop in the maxilla. Most often in the ramus and posterior mandible in older patients.

Q23. Multilocular appearance of simple bone cyst is due to:

Ans. This appearance is the result of pronounced scalloping of the endosteal surface of either the buccal or the lingual plates.

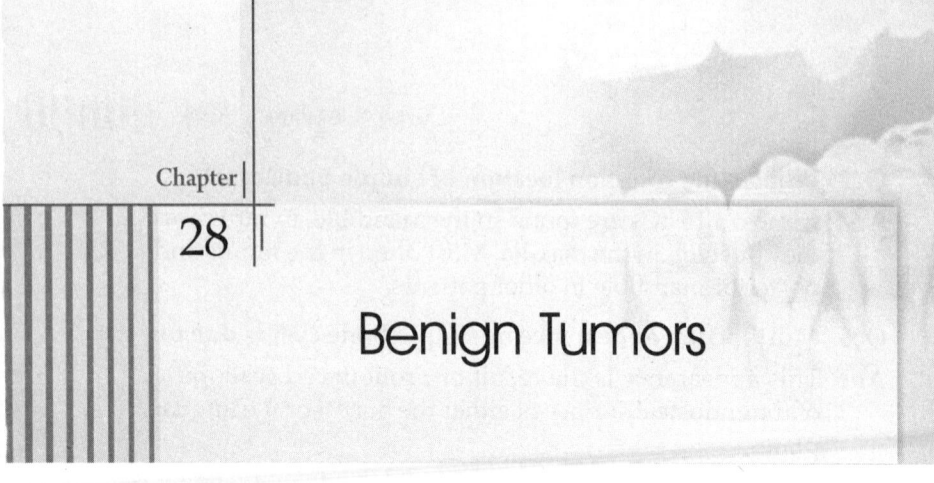

Chapter

28

Benign Tumors

Benign Tumors of the Jaws
Definition

a. Benign tumors are a well differentiated structure which may be typical of tissue origin and shows progressive and slow rate of growth.

b. *Hamartoma* are abnormal new growths (proliferation) of tissues in its usual location that cease growing along with the tissues of the associated parts.

c. *Hyperplasia* is enlargement caused by an increase in the number of cells, and the tissue in a normal arrangement.

d. *Neoplasms* are tumors that continue to grow indefinitely. It is as an abnormal mass of tissue the growth of which exceeds and is unco-ordinated with that of normal tissue and persists in some excessive manner after cessation of stimulus which evoked the change.

e. *Hypertrophy-enlargement* caused by an increase in the size of the cells.

f. *Teratoma* are neoplasms composed of a mixture of tissues, more than one of which exhibits neoplastic proliferation.

Q1. Enumerate common radiographic features of benign tumors.

Ans. They can be explained as:

Location: They have specific siterelated to origin. Odontogenic tumors occur in the alveolar process above

170

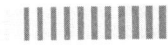

inferior alveolar canal. Vascular or neural tumor originate inside the mandibular canal.

Periphery and shape: Borders are smooth, well-defined usually and sometimes corticated. Tumor can also show a thin radiolucent band which is a soft tissue capsule.

Internal structure: May be completely radiolucent or radiopaque or combination.

Effects on surrounding structure: They are slow growing which lead to changes in bone. They exert pressure on neighbouring structures. Displaces adjacent teeth or cortices. Sometimes resorption of roots can occur.

Read: Classify benign tumors of the jaws.

Odontogenic tumors
- Epithelial or ectodermal origin
  - Ameloblastoma
  - Calcifying epithelial odontogenic tumors
- Mesenchymal or mesodermal origin
  - Cementoma (periapical cemental dysplasia)
  - Cementoblastoma (true cementoma)
  - Central cementifying fibroma
  - Florid osseous dysplasia (FOD)
  - Central odontogenic fibroma
  - Peripheral odontogenic fibroma
- Mixed tissue origin
  - Ameloblastic fibro-odontoma
  - Ameloblastic odontoma
  - Odontogenic fibroma
  - Odontogenic myxoma
  - Odontoma
    i. Compound
    ii. Complex composite
- Developmental malformation
  - Dens invaginatus (dilated odontome)
  - Dens evaginatus

Nonodontogenic tumors

- Epithelial tissue origin
  - Papiloma
  - Keratocanthoma
- Connective tissue origin
  - Fibroma of bone
    - i. Central fibroma
    - ii. Ossifying fibroma (fibro-osteoma)
    - iii. Fibroid epulis
  - Epulis
  - Pregnancy tumor
  - Benign giant cell tumor
  - Desmoplastic fibroma
  - Myxoma
  - Myxofibroma
  - Aneurysmal bone cyst
- Adipose tissue origin
  - Lipoma
  - Angiolipoma
- Cartilage tissue origin
  - Chondroma
  - Osteochondroma
    - i. Central
    - ii. Peripheral
- Bone tissue origin
  - Osteoma
  - Benign osteoblastoma
  - Torus
    - i. Palatinus
    - ii. Mandibularis

iii. Exostosis

iv. Enostoses

- Vascular tissue origin
  - Hemangioma of bone (cavernous haemangioa)
  - Hereditary hemorrhagic telengiectasia (Rendu-Osler-Weber syndrome)
- Neural tissue origin
  - Traumatic neuroma
  - Neurofibroma
  - Neuroblastoma
- Muscle tissue origin
  - Leiomyoma
  - Rhabdomyoma

Q2. Characteristics of benign tumors:

Ans. a. **Ameloblastoma**

Small loculations	– Honey comb appearance
Large loculations	– Soap bubble appearance

b. Calcifying epithelial Odontogenic tumor/ Pindborg tumor — Driven snow appearance

c. Odontogenic myxoma – Tennis racket appearance

d. Cementoblastoma – Wheel scope appearance appearance

e. Central hemangioma
  - Sunray appearance
  - Honey comb appearance
  - Serpiginous shape of inferior alveolar canal

Bone Diseases

Diseases of Bone Manifested in the Jaws

Q1. Define fibro-osseous lesion.

Ans. Fibro-osseous lesions are lesion in which there is replacement of normal bone by a tissue composed of the collagen fibers and fibroblasts containing varying amounts of mineralized substance like bone or cementum.

Q2. Classify fibro-osseous lesions of the jaw.

Ans. According to Waldron, fibro-osseous lesions are classified as;

1. Fibrous dysplasia
   - Arising in the toothbearing areas, predominantly periodontal in origin.
     i. Nonhereditary
        - Periapical cemento-osseous dysplasia
        - Focal cemento-osseous dysplasia
        - Florid cemento-osseous dysplasia
     ii. Hereditary
        Familial gigantiform cementoma
2. Fibro-osseous neoplasm
   - Cementifying fibroma
   - Ossifying fibroma
   - Cemento-ossifying fibroma
   - Juvenile ossifying fibroma
3. Cherubism

Q3. Radiographic appearaces of fibrous dysplasia.

Ans. 1. *Peau d'orange or orange peel:* Alternating areas of granular density and radiolucency resembling the peel of the orange.

2. *Whorled type:* Whorled finger print appearance.

3. Diffuse sclerotic type: Homogenous radiopaque areas

4. *Pagetoid type*: Alternating areas of opacity and lucency, similar to Paget's disease.

5. *Chalky type*: Dense radio-opacity

6. *Ground glass appearance*

Q4. What are radiographic appearaces of ossifying fibroma?

Ans. • Mixed radiolucent radiopaque lesion with radiolucent capsule.

• Internally, it shows **Wispy, flocculent pattern**.

• It causes displacement of teeth and inferior alveolar canal, with expansion of the outer cortical plates, which may be displaced and thinned but remain intact.

• Lamina dura of the involved teeth is missing with resorption of the teeth.

Q5. What is radiographic appearace of cherubism?

Ans. • Bilateral multilocular appearance is common.

• Expansion of the lesions posteriorly into the ramus and anteriorly into the body of the mandible.

• Inferior alveolar canal may be displaced.

• Maxillary lesions enlarge at the expense of the sinus.

• There is displacement of numerous teeth, prior to calcification **Floating teeth appearance**.

Q6. What is radiographic appearace of aneurysmal bone cyst?

Ans. • It is multilocular radiolucency, affecting posterior part of the jaws, **soap bubble appearance**.

• Expansion of the buccal and lingual cortical plates, causing *ballooning* or blowing out of the cortices.

• Septa may be seen within the lesion.

- The involved teeth may be tilted, bodily displaced or can be associated with external root resorption.

Q7. What is radiographic appearace of central giant cell granuloma?

Ans.
- It is seen as a solitary unilocular or multilocular lesion, with well-defined margins without cortication
- Located anterior to molars (as osteoclasts are anterior to molars)
- Internally, it shows granular pattern of calcification, organized into wispy septa giving **honeycomb appearance.**
- As it grows it causes bossing of the buccal cortex.
- Displacement of adjacent teeth, tooth buds and resorption may occur.
- The lamina dura of affected teeth is usually missing .
- The inferior alveolar canal is displaced inferiorly.

Q8. What is radiographic appearace of hyperparathyroidism?

Ans. They are as follows:
- **Metastatic calcification:** Ectopic calcification in soft tissue
- **Subperiosteal erosion:** Subperiosteal erosion of the bone, especially of the middle phalanges generalised. Loss of the lamina dura in jaws
- **Osteitis fibrosa generalisata (cystica):** Osteitis fibrosa lesions often appears cyst like areas on radiographs
- **Jaw bone changes:** The complete maxilla and the mandible are usually involved. The rarefaction may be of homogeneous nature in which normal trabecular pattern is lost and replaced by a granular or ground glass appearnce. The teeth may be mobile. There is generalized loss of lamina dura.
- **Brown giant cell lesions: Unilocular or multilocular** radiolucencies

Q9. What is radiographic appearace of florid osseous dysplasia?

Ans. • The radio-paque masses vary in size and shape that gives appearance of **generalized radio-pacities** (cotton wool).

• Well-defined radiolucent rims can be seen surrounding the masses.

• The lesion matures through the mixed stage to radiopaque stage.

• Root clubbing with *hypercementosis* may be seen.

Q10. What is radiographic appearace of osteoporosis?

Ans. • Radiographic changes in osteoporosis can be described as a decrease in density of the bone; specially a loss of the normal trabecular pattern and thinning of cortex occur.

• In jaws there is **generalized rarefaction** of bone.

• The lamina dura is lost in severe cases.

Q11. What is radiographic appearace of osteopetrosis?

Ans. • Increase density of entire skeleton resulting in diffuse homogeneous symmetrically sclerotic appearance of all bones.

• The normal landmarks are lost in dense, diffuse radio-opacity.

• The bone may appear so dense that the roots of the teeth are obscured.

• The lamina dura is often lost in overall density.

Q12. Classify bone diseases.

Ans.   i. Developmental
  • Solitary bone cyst
  • Cherubism
    Reactive/reparative
  • Central (intraosseous)
  • Garre's osteomyelitis

- Sclerosing osteomyelitis
  - a. Focal
  - b. Diffuse
- Central giant cell granuloma
- Periapical cemental dysplasia
- Aneurysmal bone cyst
- Peripheral (extraosseous)
- Peripheral giant cell granuloma

ii. **Neoplasm**
- Osteoid steoma
- Osteoblastoma
- Benign cementoblastoma

iii. **Endocrinal/Metabolic**
- Brown's tumor of hyperparathyroidism

iv. **Unknown etiology**
- Fibrous dysplasia (monostotic and polyostotic)
- Paget's disease.

Malignant Diseases

Q1. What are the general clinical characteristic features of malignant tumors affecting the jaws?

Ans.
- It may affect any age or gender
- Pain and rapid growth or ulceration or swelling of the jaw
- Malodor, indurated lesion with sometimes clinical bone exposure
- displaced or loosened teeth
- Sensory or motor nerve function impairment
- Lymphadenopathy (hard lymph node)
- Weight loss, dysguesia, dysphagia, haemorrhage can be present
- Dyspnoea, fatigue, loss of apetite, fever are other associated symptoms which patient can present.

Q2. What are the common radiographic features of malignant lesions of the jaw?

Ans. They can be described as:

Location—varies as per the site of involvement.

Periphery and shape
- **Finger like extensions** of the tumor
- **Bays and promontories** or bay in bay appearance.
- Shape of the lesion is *irregular*.
- Peripheral lesions show cupped out appearance
- *Ragged borders*

Internal structure—if residual islands of bone are present, they give mixed RL-RO appearance. Internal trabeculae are destroyed. Usually seen as an ill defined osteolytic lesion with lack of cortication.

- Effect on surrounding structures –
  - Widening of PDLs or loss of lamina dura
  - Destruction of mandibular canal.
  - Lesion may destroy sinus boundaries, cortices, follicular cortices and inferior border of mandible.
  - Displaced or loosened teeth give *floating tooth appearance* on radiographs.
  - Periosteal bone reaction can be seen as *onion skin appearance*.

Q3. Which tumors induce bone formation instead of bone destruction?

Ans. Metastatic prostate and breast lesions

Q4. Which malignant tumor is associated with bone deposition than resorption?

Ans. Osteosarcoma

Q5. Which two features together are highly suggestive of malignancy?

Ans. Evidence of destruction of cortical bone with adjacent soft tissue mass

Q6. Which characteristic root resorption is seen in malignancy?

Ans. Spiked root resorption

Q7. Root resorption is common in which tumors?

Ans. Sarcomas and multiple myeloma

Q8. Hair-on-end or sunburst appearance is seen in:

Ans. 1. Osteosarcoma
2. Ewing's sarcoma
3. Fibrosarcoma
4. Non-Hodgkin's lymphoma
5. Burkitt lymphoma

6. Metastatic tumor of the jaw
7. Prostate
8. Neuroblastoma
9. Hemangioma
10. Sickle cell anemia
11. Thalassemia

Q9. Which malignant tumor presents with soap bubble/ honeycomb appearance?

Ans. Mucoepidermoid carcinoma

Q10. Which two bone lesions are commonly associated with osteosarcoma?

Ans. Fibrous dysplasia and Paget's disease

Q11. Radiographic features of osteosarcoma:

Ans. • Codman's triangle (also seen in chondrosarcoma, fibrosarcoma)
   • Garrington's sign is thickening of PDL space of involoved teeth due to infiltration of malignant cells.
   • Moth-eaten appearance/salt-pepper appearance
   • Laminar periosteal new bone formation/onion skin appearance

Q12. Which lesions share radiographic characteristics with osteosarcoma?

Ans. Ewing's sarcoma, solitary plasmacytoma, osteomyelitis.

Q13. Moth-eaten appearance/salt-pepper appearance is seen in:

Ans. Osteosarcoma, chondrosarcoma, osteomyelitis.

Q14. Other name for Ewing's sarcoma:

Ans. Round cell tumor/endothelial myeloma.

Q15. Laminar periosteal new bone formation/onion skin appearance seen in:

Ans. Ewing's sarcoma, non-Hodgkin's lymphoma

Q16. Which tumor is known as great imitator and why?

Ans. Central hemangioma due to many radiographic appearance is called great imitator.

Q17. Radiographic features of multiple myeloma.

Ans. Its radiographic features are punched out radiolucency. (well-defined without corticated borders)

In this malignancy teeth appear too opaque/stand out conspicuously from their osteopenic background.

Q18. Punched out radiolucency is seen in which lesion?

Ans. 1. Multiple myeloma (well-defined without corticated borders)

2. Punched out lesions are seen clinically in ANUG.

Paranasal Sinus Diseases

Q1. Classify disorders of paranasal sinuses.

Ans.

1. Traumatic	Fractures
2. Infective	Sinusitis (acute or chronic), osteomyelitis, tuberculosis, actinomycosis, etc.
3. Cysts (intrinsic or extrinsic)	Mucous retention cyst, mucocele, radicular or kerato-cyst
4. Neoplasm	Ameloblastoma, cementoma, antral polyp, exostosis, enostosis, osteoma, chondroma squamous cell CA, etc.
5. Metabolic and endocrinal	Fibrous dysplasia, cherubism. Paget's disease
6. Calcifications	Antroliths
7. Syndromes	Treacher Collin's syndrome, Crouzon's syndrome

Q2. How is the radiographic appearance of normal paranasal sinuses?

Ans. The antrum appears as a radiolucent cavity in the maxilla, with well-defined, dense, corticated radiopaque margins or walls. The internal bony septa and blood vessels canals in the walls produce their own shadows.

Q3. What are the different imaging techniques to visualize sinuses?

Ans. IOPA radiograph, maxillary lateral occlusal view, OPG helps to visualize major areas of sinus with visualization

of inferior, posterior, and anteromedial walls. Other views to support information obtained from above radiographs are; Waters' view, CBCT, CT including MRI (soft tissue).

Q4. Which imaging modalities can help to visualize sinus?

Ans. • Panoramic radiograph shows greater internal structure and parts of the inferior, posterior and anteromedial walls.

• Caldwell's posteroanterior view shows frontal sinus, ethmoidal air cells, nasal cavity and superior portion of the maxillary antrum.

• Waters' view shows the roof, medial walls

• Lateral skull view shows the sphenoidal and maxillary sinuses the anterior and superior walls. Submento-vertex shows lateral and posterior borders of the maxillary sinus

• Computed tomography gives 3D view of the disease

• Scintigraphy, in case of extension of the antral carcinoma to involve bone, the osteoblastic response produced is clearly evident in the delayed phase of a radionuclide bone scan.

• Ultrasound helps in distinguishing normal sinuses, chronically inflamed sinus or soft tissue pathologies

• Magnetic resonance imaging. It helps to delineate soft tissue in the sinus.

Q5. Radiographic features of various disorders of sinus.

Ans.

S. no	Disease	Radiographic features
1.	Mucositis	Noncorticated radiopaque area/band along the lining
2.	Maxillary sinusitis	• Thickening of sinus mucosa • Sinus becomes radiopaque • Thickening can be uniform or polypoid • In case of fluid accumulations—horizontal/straight line • Chronic—persistent radiopacification

(Contd.)

(Contd.)

S. no	Disease	Radiographic features
3.	Pseudocyst	• Well-defined, non-corticated, smooth, dome-shaped, sessile radiopaque homogeneous mass with no effect on surrounding structures.
4.	Polyp	• Thickened mucosal lining • Destruction of bone
5.	Mucocele	• Change in the shape of sinus—more circular. • Internally—uniform radiopacity • Displaces margins of sinus and expands the bone • Teeth may get displaced, resorbed roots
6.	Neoplasms benign	• Homogeneous radiopaque mass of soft tissue density. • Sharp defined margins usually • Bone destruction if present is due to pressure due to tumor
7.	Malignancy	• Internal radiopacity with destructions of walls as it grows • Irregular radiolucent areas in the surrounding bone. • Irregular widening of PDL

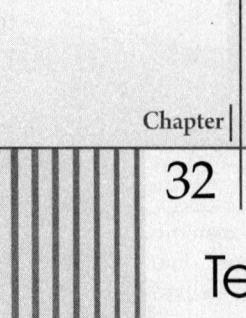

Temporomandibular Joint Disorders

Q1. Name various imaging methods for TMJ.

Ans. • OPG
  • Transpharyngeal view
  • Transorbital view
  • Transcranrial view
  • CBCT
  • MRI
  • CT
  • Arthrography
  • Arthroscopy

Q2. What are the main indication of transpharyngeal radiography?

Ans. a. To investigate the presence of joint disease like osteoarthritis and rheumatoid arthritis
  b. To investigate pathological conditions affecting the condylar head, including cyst or tumors
  c. Fractures of neck and head of condyle

Q3. What are the indications of MRI for TMJ disorder.

Ans. a. When diagnosis of internal disc derangements is in doubt
  b. For preoperative assessment of disc.

Q4. Which diagnostic information CT can provide?

Ans. a. The shape of the condyle and condition of articulating surfaces
  b. The condition of the glenoid fossa and eminence

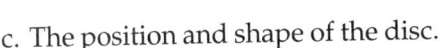

c. The position and shape of the disc.

d. The integrity of the disc and its soft tissue attachments.

e. Condyle head abnormalities.

Q5. What are the indications of arthrography?

Ans. a. In cases of limited mouth opening of unknown etiology

b. Long history of locking of jaw

c. Chronic TMJ pain.

Q6. Enumerate radiographic features of following TMJ disorders:

Ans. a. MPDS—no features unless and until bony component is involved.

b. Internal derangement—MRI can help to show disc position and disc movement

c. Osteoarthritis—flattening of head of condyle, subchondral sclerosis, osteophyte formation, Ely's cysts.

d. Rheumatoid arthritis—erosion and destruction of articular surface of head of condyle, hollowing of glenoid fossa, **sharpened pencil appearance** condyle bilateral involvement usually.

e. Alkylosis—little or no evidence of joint space, bony Union of condyle and glenoid fossa and may be associated with condyle hypoplasia or mandibular under-development. Prominent antegonial notch can also be evident.

f. Dislocation—condyle is located anterior or superior to the boundaries of articular eminence.

Q7. Which are specialized views of TMJ?

Ans. The views are:

• Transcranial and transpharyngeal provide lateral aspect of condyle

• Transorbital depicts mediolateral aspect of TMJ in frontal plane

• Transpharyngeal (taken in open mouth position) depicts medial aspect of condyle.

Soft Tissue Calcifications and Ossifications

Q1. Classify soft tissue calcification.

Ans. Heterotrophic calcifications

   A. Dystrophic calcifications, e.g. calcified lymph nodes, dystrophic calcification in the tonsils, arterial calcification, calcified atherosclerotic plaque.

   B. Idiopathic calcifications, e.g. sialoliths, phleboliths, rhinolith/antrolith

   C. Metastatic calcifications

Heterotrophic ossifications: Ossification of the stylohyoid ligament, osteoma cutis, myositis ossificans.

Q2. What are the general radiographic features of soft tissue calcifications?

Ans.
- Soft tissue calcifications can be seen in IOPA as well as in panoramic radiographs.
- Calcifications adjacent to bone are sometimes difficult to diagnose but additional or another radiographic view at right angles can give useful information.
- Knowledge of the soft tissue anatomy, such as the position of lymph nodes, stylohyoid ligament, blood vessels, laryngeal cartilages, the major ducts of the salivary glands are important to interpret the anatomical location, number, distribution and shape of the calcification.
- Calcifications can be considered as differential diagnosis for solitary radiopacities not contacting teeth, multiple separate radiopacities or false periapical radiopacities.

Notes

Concept	Event Year	Inventor
Discovery of X-ray	1895	W C Roentgen
First dental radiograph	1896	O Walkhoff
First paper on dangers of X-radiation	1901	WH Rollins
Introduction of bisecting technique	1904	WA Price
First X-ray tube	1913	WD Coolidge
Concept of paralleling technique	1920	F McCormack
First dental X-ray machine	1923	Vector X-ray corporation of Chicago

- Properties of X-rays
    1. They travel in a straight line.
    2. They travel through space and matter.
    3. They travel with the speed of visible light, i.e. 1,86,000 miles/second.
    4. They are invisible to eye.
    5. They cannot be reflected, refracted or deflected.
    6. They do not possess any charge
    7. They do not require medium for propagation.
    8. They are electromagnetic radiations having wavelength between 10 Å and 0.01 Å.

9. Penetration, absorption, ionization, fluorescence are few diagnostic properties of X-rays.

- Hard and soft rays—X-rays range in energy from 100 eV to 100 keV (below 0.2–0.1 nm wavelength). Hard X-rays are those with photon energies greater than 5–10 keV. Soft X-rays are those with lower energy.

A. Name pulpoperiapical radiolucencies/differential diagnosis.

1. Periapical lesions
   - Periapical granuloma
   - Radicular cyst
   - Scar
   - Chronic and acute dentoalveolar abscesses
   - Surgical defect
   - Osteomyelitis
2. Dentigerous cyst
3. Periapical cemento-osseous
   - Dysplasia (periapical cementoma)
4. Periodontal disease.

B. Enlist few pericoronal radiolucencies.

1. Pericornol or follicular space
2. Dentigerous cyst
3. Unicystic (mural)
4. Ameloblastoma
5. Adenomatoid odontogenic tumor
6. Calcifying odotogenic cyst or tumor'
7. Ameloblastic fibroma

C. Enlist multiple separate radiolucent lesions.

- Multiple cysts or granulomas
- Basal cell nevus syndrome

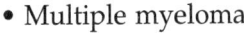

- Multiple myeloma
- Metastatic carcinoma
- Langerhans' cell disease

D. Which are the conditions causing generalized rarefactions of the jaws.

1. Hyperparathyroidism
   - Primary
   - Secondary
   - Tertiary
2. Osteoporosis
   - Postmenopausal and senile osteoporosis
   - Drug induced osteoporosis
   - Osteoporosis of Cushing's syndrome
   - Osteoporosis of malnutritional states
3. Osteomalacia
4. Hereditary hemolytic anemia
   - Thalassemia
   - Sickle cell anemia
5. Leukemia
6. Langerhans' cell disease
7. Paget's disease (early stage)
8. Multiple myeloma (late stage)

E. Name few lesions appearing as periapical radiopacities

1. Condensing or sclerosing osteitis
2. Periapical idiopathic osteosclerosis
3. Periapical or focal cemento-osseous dysplasia
4. Unerupted succedaneous teeth
5. Foreign bodies
6. Hypercementosis

False periapical radiopacities

1. Anatomic structures
2. Impacted teeth, supernumerary teeth, and compound odontomas

F. Name the conditions giving appearance of multiple separate radiopacities

- Tori and exostoses
- Multiple retained roots
- Multiple socket sclerosis
- Multiple periapical or focal cemento-osseous dysplasia
- Multiple periapical condensing osteitis
- Multiple embedded or impacted teeth

G. Name the conditions giving appearance of generalised radiopacities

- Florid cemento-osseous dysplasia
- Paget's disease—mature stage
- Osteopetrosis

H. Name few interradicular radiolucencies.

Anatomic	*Pathologic*
Tooth crypt	Furcation involvement
Mental foramen and canal	Traumatic bone cyst
Lateral fossa	Lateral radicular cyst
Maxillary sinus	Other odontogenic cyst

I. Name the conditions giving appearance of multilocular lesion

- Ameloblastoma
- Cherubism
- Odontogenic myxoma
- OKC
- ABC
- CGCG

J. Name the conditions giving mixed radiopaque radiolucent appearance

- PCOD
- Cemento-ossifying fibroma
- Odontome
- AOT
- COC
- CEOT

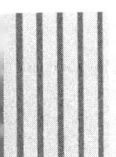

References

- Burket's Oral Medicine. Diagnosis and Treatment, 10th edition. Lester William Burket, Martin S. Greenberg, Michael Glick. People's Medical Publishing House, USA, 2003.
- Burket's Oral Medicine, 11th edition. Martin Greenberg, Michael *Glick, Jonathan A. Ship.* People's Medical Publishing House, USA, 2008.
- Burket's Oral Medicine. 12th edition. Michael Glick. Shelton, Connecticut : People's Medical Publishing House, USA, 2015.
- Burket's Oral Medicine. Diagnosis and Treatment, 9th edition. Malcolm A. Lynch, Vernon John Brightman, Martin S. Greenberg. Lippincott, 1994.
- Concise Oral medicine. HR. Umarji, 2009. CBS Publishers & Distributors Pvt. Ltd.
- Medical Problems in Dentistry, 4th Edition. Crispian Scully and Roderick A. Cawson, 1998
- White SC, Pharoah MJ. Oral Radiology: Principles and Interpretation, First South Asia ed. New Delhi, Mosby; 2014.
- Wood NK, Good PW. Differential diagnosis of oral maxillofacial lesions. 5th ed. St. Louis : Mosby; 1997.
- Karjodkar FR. Essentials of oral and maxillofacial Radiology, New Delhi : Jaypee; 2014.
- White SC, Pharoah MJ. Oral radiology principles and Interpretation. 6th ed. St. Louis: Mosby; 2009.
- White SC, Pharaoh MJ. oral radiology principles and Interpretation. 5th ed. St. Louis: Mosby; 2004.
- Haring JM, Havertown LJ. Dental Radiography Principal and techniques. 3rd ed. St. Louis: Squander's;
- Whites E, Cawson RA. Essentials of Dental radiography and radiology. 2nd ed. New York US: Churchill Livingston.
- Whites E, Cawson RA. Essentials of Dental Radiography and Radiology. 4th ed. London: Churchill Livingston.
- Langland OE, Langlais RP. Principles of Dental imaging. Pennsylvania: Edward, Brothers; 1997.